T0200662

EMBODIED
WISDOM

Also by MOSHE FELDENKRAIS

Body and Mature Behavior:
A Study of Anxiety, Sex, Gravitation, and Learning

The Potent Self: A Study of Spontaneity and Compulsion

Awareness Through Movement

Body Awareness as Healing Therapy: The Case of Nora

The Elusive Obvious

The Master Moves

Practical Unarmed Combat

Judo: The Art of Defense and Attack

Higher Judo: Groundwork

EMBODIED WISDOM

The Collected Papers of
MOSHE FELDENKRAIS

Moshe Feldenkrais

Foreword by David Zemach-Bersin

Edited by Elizabeth Beringer

Somatic Resources
San Diego, California

North Atlantic Books
Berkeley, California

Published by
Somatic Resources
3680 Sixth Avenue
San Diego, California 92103

and
North Atlantic Books
Huichin, unceded Ohlone land
aka Berkeley, California

Cover photo by Lionel Delevingne
Cover and book design by Suzanne Albertson
Printed in Canada

Photos © 2010. See page 221–222 for photo credits.
Photos on 36, 40, 61, and 65 are used with permission from the International Feldenkrais Federation.

Photographs © by Michael Wolgensinger appear courtesy of the Wolgensinger archive, leawolgensinger@simplicity.ch.

"Bodily Expression," *Somatics,* Vol. 6, No. 4, Spring/Summer 1988. Translated from the French by Thomas Hanna. "Bodily Expression (Conclusion)," *Somatics,* Vol. 7, No. 1, Autumn/Winter 1988–89. "On the Primacy of Hearing," *Somatics,* Vol. 1, No. 1, Autumn 1976. "Man and the World," *Somatics,* Vol. 2, No. 2, Spring 1979. Reprinted by permission of *Somatics* magazine.

Feldenkrais, Moshe. Edited and translated by Kelly Morris, "Image, Movement, and Actor: Restoration of Potentiality." *TDR: The Drama Review* volume 10: number 3, T31, Spring, 1966. Reprinted by permission of the publisher. Rotté, Joanne. "Feldenkrais Revisited: Tension, Talent, and the Legacy of Childhood." Courtesy of Joanne Rotté.

Embodied Wisdom: The Collected Papers of Moshe Feldenkrais is sponsored and published by North Atlantic Books, an educational nonprofit based in the unceded Ohlone land Huichin (*aka* Berkeley, CA) that collaborates with partners to develop cross-cultural perspectives; nurture holistic views of art, science, the humanities, and healing; and seed personal and global transformation by publishing work on the relationship of body, spirit, and nature.

North Atlantic Books' publications are distributed to the US trade and internationally by Penguin Random House Publisher Services. For further information, visit our website at www.northatlanticbooks.com.

Feldenkrais®, Feldenkrais Method®, Functional Integration®, Awareness Through Movement®, and Guild Certified *Feldenkrais* Practitioner® are service marks of the *Feldenkrais* GUILD® of North America.

Library of Congress Cataloging-in-Publication Data
Feldenkrais, Moshé, 1904–1984.
  Embodied wisdom : the collected papers of Moshé Freldenkrais / Moshé Freldenkrais ; edited by Elizabeth Beringer.
    p. ; cm.
  Includes bibliographical references.
  ISBN 978-1-55643-906-3
1. Feldenkrais method. I. Beringer, Elizabeth. II. Title. [DNLM: 1. Feldenkrais, Moshé, 1904–1984. 2. Psychophysiology—Collected Works. 3. Psychophysiology—Interview. 4. Body Image—Collected Works. 5. Body Image—Interview. 6. Motor Activity—Collected Works. 7. Motor Activity—Interview. 8. Self Concept—Collected Works. 9. Self Concept—Interview. WL 103 F312e 2010]
  RC489.F44F4423 2010
  616.80092'2—dc22   2010020233

8 9 10 11 12 MQ 24 23 22

This book includes recycled material and material from well-managed forests. North Atlantic Books is committed to the protection of our environment. We print on recycled paper whenever possible and partner with printers who strive to use environmentally responsible practices.

Dedicated to all the *Feldenkrais* practitioners worldwide who are putting Moshe Feldenkrais's ideas into action.

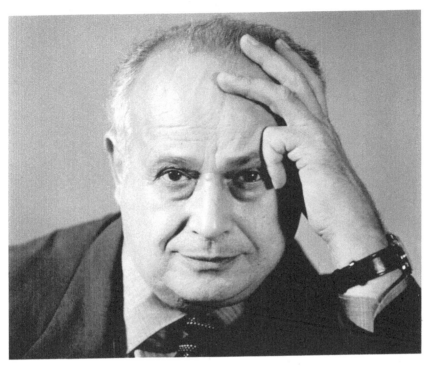

Moshe Feldenkrais 1904–1984

Contents

Foreword

I believe that the unity of mind and body is an objective reality. They are not just parts somehow related to each other, but an inseparable whole while functioning. A brain without a body could not think ... the muscles themselves are part and parcel of our higher functions.
MOSHE FELDENKRAIS, from the article "Mind and Body," 1964

Movement is life. Life is a process. Improve the quality of the process and you improve the quality of life itself.
MOSHE FELDENKRAIS, from *Awareness Through Movement*, 1973

MOSHE FELDENKRAIS WAS ONE OF THE TWENTIETH CENTURY's most original and integrative thinkers. Along with such seminal figures as Ida Rolf, Heinrich Jacoby, F. M. Alexander, and Elsa Gindler, Feldenkrais is considered one of the founders of the field that is today called Somatics. The pieces included in *Embodied Wisdom: The Collected Papers of Moshe Feldenkrais* were originally published in independent journals between 1964 and 1998. A testament to the prescience of Feldenkrais's ideas is the fact that many of the concepts presented in this volume are as important, generative, and radical today as they were when they were first articulated. In these remarkable articles and interviews, Feldenkrais provides us with some of the most cogent and sophisticated arguments ever made for the biological and functional unity of the mind and body.

During most of the twentieth century, the dominant medical and academic model of the brain was that our habits are fixed or hard-wired, that each area of the brain has specialized, pre-determined functions, and that every day of our adulthood, our brain loses both neurons and the ability to learn new skills. In books, articles, and lectures from 1949 to 1981, Moshe Feldenkrais strongly challenged this point of view, not simply the theory behind it, but in practice, by developing innovative exercises and clinical applications that effectively demonstrated that—even when damaged—the brain has the ability to quickly change, and to learn new skills and recover lost functions.

Today, a new paradigm is taking hold in neuroscience, psychology, and rehabilitation: the concept of brain plasticity, or neuroplasticity, which posits that throughout our entire life span, our brain has the capacity to modify its organization and responses through experience and learning. If Feldenkrais were alive, he would find today's research supporting neuroplasticity a sweet validation.

In April 1973, when I first observed Dr. Feldenkrais working, it was clear that he believed in each person's capacity to learn and change. Feldenkrais was teaching a month-long seminar in Berkeley, where I was a pre-med student at the University of California. After my regular courses, I would sneak into the classroom where he was teaching. What I saw there was extraordinary.

Each day, as part of his seminar, Feldenkrais would work for one hour with a middle-aged man named Edward, who had severe spastic cerebral palsy. On my first day observing, Edward's speech was nearly impossible to understand, his arms were hyper-flexed and pulled up near his chest, his hands twisted inward, and he moved slowly with a halting, effortful gait. Since early childhood, Edward had received the best physical therapy and medical attention possible.

Edward would lie on a firm, padded table while Feldenkrais "worked" with him, gently moving him in mysterious ways, but clearly with great care, dexterity, intelligence, and deliberateness. Feldenkrais explained that he was using gentle, functionally oriented movement to help Edward's nervous system learn to change the messages it was sending to his musculature. After a few weeks, Edward's improvement was nothing short of miraculous. His speech became easy to understand, his arms rested by his sides, and his walking was much more comfortable and efficient. In short, his entire way of organizing himself had changed. I could not understand how this "healing" had occurred, yet I was incredibly excited and moved by what I had seen. By the end of the year, I would graduate from Berkeley, travel to Tel Aviv, Israel, and knock on Dr. Feldenkrais's door, eager to understand how he had created the "transformation" that I had witnessed in Berkeley.

The revolutionary concepts that served as the theoretical framework for Feldenkrais's work with Edward are explored in *Embodied Wisdom: The*

Collected Papers of Moshe Feldenkrais. These unique writings have relevance in domains as diverse as neuroscience and theater, psychology and dance, physical therapy and music, education and rehabilitation, and infant development and athletic performance.

This volume presents Feldenkrais's most concise and cohesive statements on the theory behind his work, written in a warm and conversational tone. In addition, you will find interviews in which Feldenkrais discusses the early history of judo in Europe, and the application of his ideas to acting, and a transcript of an illuminating conversation between Feldenkrais and noted Israeli scientist Aharon Katzir.

Originally a scientist working at the cutting edge of physics, Feldenkrais was a well-read and wide-ranging thinker. In these articles and interviews he draws from insights in physics, biology, embryology, psychology, semantics, and neurology, and makes speculative leaps about the brain and learning that have been verified by contemporary neuroscience. You will find that Feldenkrais almost always lets you in on his thinking process, allowing you to share in his logic, which often leads to surprising conclusions. At times he takes a highly abstract or theoretical idea and turns it like a Rubik's Cube in order to help us to see it from every possible angle. And, he nearly always shows us the everyday, concrete implications of the concept. Some might call his writing style Socratic or even Talmudic, and these may both be true, but it also represents Feldenkrais's background as a rigorous scientist. This is especially in evidence when he asks us to join him in thinking with a hyper clarity as he deconstructs such common, everyday words or concepts as "consciousness" or "thinking" or "self-image" or "energy" or "fulfillment." In these moments, we are treated to a classically educated, keen analytic mind, asking that we define our terms precisely, and demonstrating how this attention to specificity often leads us down paths we would not have otherwise explored.

Common to every article and interview in this unique collection is Feldenkrais's optimism about the capacity of each one of us—no matter our circumstances or limitations—to grow, change, improve, and become a more self-determined human being. This hopeful outlook is not so much strategic, as it is founded upon the strong evidence that of our brain's one hundred billion neurons, we use only a very small percentage, leaving the rest available for learning new ways of moving, feeling, thinking, and acting.

So, how did Feldenkrais, someone who had been a physicist for more than twenty years, come to develop the skills necessary to help Edward learn to move, speak, and function more easily? Great insights often emerge out of great struggle, and as it happened, Feldenkrais personally suffered from a debilitating problem for which medicine offered no solution. In his search for an answer to his own difficulties, Feldenkrais developed some of his most important ideas.

Moshe Pinchas Feldenkrais, DSc, was born in 1904, in a small town in a part of Russia that is today the Ukraine. He had been given the middle name Pinchas in honor of his great-great-great-grandfather, Pinchas of Korets, a famous rabbi and one of the leading disciples of Rabbi Israel ben Eliezer, the founder of Hassidism, commonly known as the Baal Shem Tov.

When he was thirteen years old, fleeing anti-Semitism and pogroms, Feldenkrais traveled from Russia, by foot, to the British Mandate of Palestine. There he worked, studied, and developed an interest in self-defense techniques. In 1930, he moved to Paris to study engineering and physics at the Sorbonne. In addition to his academic work, Feldenkrais studied Japanese martial arts and was one of the first people from the West to receive a black belt in judo. His appreciation of judo was illuminated by his understanding of the physics of movement—how the laws of motion and gravity impact the mechanics of movement. In 1933, Feldenkrais began working on his doctoral degree and was part of a team of scientists at the Curie Institute conducting research and publishing early papers on nuclear fission with Nobel Prize laureate physicist Frédéric Joliot-Curie.

With the German invasion of Paris in 1940, Feldenkrais escaped to England, where he spent the war conducting military research for the British government. During this time, due to knee injuries suffered over the years, Feldenkrais found himself unable to walk without great pain and difficulty. Modern arthroscopic surgery techniques had yet to be developed, and the top English surgeons whom Feldenkrais consulted offered him little hope of improvement through medical intervention. Feldenkrais decided to try to solve his problem by himself.

With the rigor of a scientist, Feldenkrais began a study of functional anatomy, applied the laws of physics and motion to everyday human movement, and explored the process by which we originally acquire our most basic motor functions. He eventually came to a remarkable practical understanding: that learning is the primary ingredient in our formation. He thought that if he could understand how learning actually takes place, then he might be able to change old habit patterns and restore lost functions, such as his own ability to walk. This quest would change the direction of his professional life.

Unlike most other mammals, we are born with a brain that is essentially *tabula rasa* (a clean slate); that is, apart from our most basic physiological functions and drives, we are not "wired-in" at birth. For nearly everything that we are eventually able to do as adults, we need a period of apprenticeship or learning. For example, most infants need ten to fourteen months before they can walk, and before walking is possible they must first learn to roll over, sit up, crawl, stand, and so on. From Feldenkrais's point of view, every child has to independently, organically learn how to solve concrete physical problems such as gravity, stability and instability, momentum, equilibrium, and so forth.

The functions that we identify as being uniquely "human" would not emerge if we were raised in a completely isolated environment. Unlike most other species, humans need more than simply air and sustenance. We require a human social world, one in which, over time, intention and successful action develop in correspondence to fulfilling meaningful goals in a context with others.

Feldenkrais developed a point of view that gives primacy to the nervous system and movement. He makes the extremely bold proposal that it is through the medium of movement that the nervous system makes the distinctions that lead to preferences or choices for particular actions or behavioral patterns.

The advantage of a largely unwired-in nervous system to a human being is that it enables tremendous flexibility in relation to behavioral options. In other words, we can learn to adapt to an unlimited number of cultural environments, languages, climates, and so on. By the same token, if we are not hard-wired for ideal movement or posture or behaviors, then we are vulnerable to making choices that may not be the best for us. Choices we make as children may not serve our long-term interests, resulting in neuromuscular ailments such as back and neck pain, neurotic inclinations, depression, and poor self-image.

Feldenkrais began to understand that there is an inseparable relationship between our social-psychological development and our motor development. As children, our psychic-emotional patterns or behaviors and our growing movement repertoire are not only being learned concurrently, but they are realized in the moment, as an integrated whole, through the musculature. These insights are explored in Feldenkrais's first two books, *Body and Mature Behavior: A Study of Anxiety, Sex, Gravitation, and Learning* and *The Potent Self.*

> *In a perfectly matured body which has grown without great emotional disturbances, movements tend gradually to conform to the mechanical requirements of the surrounding world. The nervous system has evolved under the influence of these laws and is fitted to them. However, in our society we do, by the promise of great reward or intense punishment, so distort the even development of the system, that many acts become excluded or restricted.*
>
> MOSHE FELDENKRAIS, *Body and Mature Behavior*

Believing that the adult brain has an abundance of potential for learning, Feldenkrais asked, what are the conditions in which a nervous system—or, rather, a person—can learn most easily, most successfully? In a bold original synthesis, Feldenkrais found the answer to this question in a little-known nineteenth-century discovery in psychophysics (the precursor to modern-day experimental psychology) known as the Weber-Fechner Theorem, or The Law of Just Noticeable Difference.

In general terms, the Weber-Fechner law states that there is a constant ratio between the magnitude of a stimulus (for example, sound, light, muscular work, and so on) and the change in that stimulus that is needed for a person to notice a difference. In practical terms, what this means is that the greater the magnitude or intensity of a stimulus, the greater is the change needed in order for us to notice a difference; or conversely, as the intensity of the stimulus decreases, the order of change needed to notice a difference becomes smaller and smaller.

Feldenkrais understood that by reducing muscular effort, kinesthetic-sensory acuity is improved and it becomes possible for a person to make fine distinctions about what they are doing and to become aware of unconscious or unknown aspects of their physical organization, movement, and action.

Feldenkrais realized that his inability to walk was not simply a matter of the poor structural integrity of his knees, but also of the "way" that he walked. In other words, his learned habits of movement were contributing to his problems. This is what Feldenkrais would come to call the general problem of "faulty learning." He realized that if he could develop a practical means of applying the Weber-Fechner law with functional movement, he would have the means for optimizing the conditions for learning, improvement, and rehabilitation.

A fundamental change in the motor pattern will thereby leave thought and also feeling without anchorage in the pattern of their established routines. Habit has lost its chief support, that of the muscles, and has become more amenable to change.
    MOSHE FELDENKRAIS, *Awareness Through Movement*

Feldenkrais continued to refine his discoveries, and eventually restored his ability to walk. In the process, he developed two entirely original and distinct modalities for realizing his ideas: a one-on-one individual method eventually named *Functional Integration®*, and a group method now known as *Awareness Through Movement®*. In *Awareness Through Movement,* his discoveries were codified as highly structured self-explorations or guided learning experiments. In both modalities, fundamental or synergistic neuromuscular relationships are utilized to facilitate healthier, more efficient patterns of movement, and posture.

Feldenkrais returned to Israel in 1949, to conduct physics research at the Weizmann Institute and assume the post of director of the Electronics

Department of the Israel Defense Forces. At the same time he continued to teach his group classes and develop the practical methods to apply his findings on the mind-body relationship. Chaim Weizmann, a fellow scientist and the first president of Israel, told Feldenkrais, "There are many others in physics who understand what you understand, but there is no one else who has the insights about the body that you do." The effectiveness of Feldenkrais's work came to be so well known that he finally left the world of physics research in the mid-1950s and started a clinic to help people with a wide range of difficulties, and performing artists seeking to improve their abilities.

Feldenkrais often said that *Awareness Through Movement* and *Functional Integration* are two sides of one coin, meaning that both applications are derived from the same over-arching theory. He was constantly developing and testing both forms. Always foremost was his thesis that the nexus of learning, awareness, and movement provides the most direct means for improving a person's well-being.

Through his daily clinical work over the next thirty years, Feldenkrais developed effective, ingenious, and innovative strategies for improving or restoring nearly every human function. He worked with internationally noted actors, musicians, and dancers, such as theater directors Peter Brook and Jacques Lecoq, and musicians Yehudi Menuhin, Narciso Yepes, and Igor Markevitch, and spent so much time with his clinical practice and teaching that he published only one extensive clinical study, *The Case of Nora*. Fortunately we have nearly two hundred hours of his *Functional Integration* work on film, and in the more than one thousand experiential *Awareness Through Movement* lessons that he created, we have a written record of Feldenkrais's thinking as it developed.

Feldenkrais's first training of Practitioners of his work took place in Tel Aviv and was completed in 1971 with thirteen graduates. During the early 1970s, Feldenkrais began to teach abroad in both Europe and the United States, and well-known intellectuals and performing artists took an interest in his ideas, including: political figures David Ben-Gurion and Moshe Dayan, anthropologist Margaret Mead, neuroscientists Paul Bach-y-Rita and Karl Pribram, physiologist Elmer Green, and psychologist William Schutz. With growing international attention, Feldenkrais began his second training of Practitioners in 1975 in San Francisco with a group of sixty students. In 1980 he began his third training program in Amherst, Massachusetts, with more than 230 students from fifteen different countries. Since then, his work has continued to grow and now there are nearly ten thousand Feldenkrais Practitioners in more than forty different countries.

When I knocked, unannounced, on Feldenkrais's door in early 1974, he generously allowed me to sit in his clinic for many months, watching him work with his students. He never used the word "patient," as he thought that it put the accent on a person's pathology and he wanted the emphasis to be on their potential to learn. What I saw during those months was no less amazing than what I had observed in Berkeley the year before: a woman with multiple sclerosis being able to abandon her cane, a severely spinal cord injured American able to give up his wheelchair for crutches, a seven-year-old Israeli boy who had never been able to open his left eye learning to open and close both eyes at the same time, a German cellist who had suffered a stroke learning to use his bowing arm once again, and a young Austrian girl with cerebral palsy learning to walk. I was privileged to study with Feldenkrais until his death in Tel Aviv in 1984, and find myself, still today, fascinated and engaged by his ideas.

The legacy of Dr. Moshe Feldenkrais has the potential to help millions of people who suffer from aches, pains, movement difficulties, and debilitating neurological problems, as well as performing artists and athletes hoping to improve their abilities. In this foreword, I have touched upon only a few of the implications and applications of Feldenkrais's work. I believe that areas such as physical medicine, physical therapy, education, and psychology have much to learn from Feldenkrais's theories and methods. I hope that the publication of this important and long overdue book will help bring his uniquely original and innovative ideas the recognition and the critical analysis they so deserve, and that readers will appreciate this small volume, which is so large in outlook and vision.

DAVID ZEMACH-BERSIN
Feldenkrais Institute of New York
and Doylestown, Pennsylvania
March 2010

Editor's Introduction

THE LAST BOOK WRITTEN BY MOSHE FELDENKRAIS was enticingly titled *The Elusive Obvious*. The title refers to how the importance of our learned self-organization is elusive until the change of perspective suggested by Feldenkrais makes it obvious. The shift from elusive to obvious would also be an apt description for this book project. When the idea came to me to publish this collection of articles, it was immediately obvious that this book made sense. The articles have never been generally available, even though they include some of the most accessible of Feldenkrais's writings. The book gathers all of Feldenkrais's articles and interviews published* in English related to the *Feldenkrais Method®*. They span the period between 1964 and 1981. Although some of the interviews were published later, all the actual interviews took place within this time frame. I have added brief histories to each piece and introduced the editors and interviewers when relevant. I have also added notes throughout the articles to give additional background material.

In the writings collected here, Feldenkrais refers to many individuals, sometimes famous politicians, artists, or scientists, other times figures from his era, who would have been known to the particular subculture he was teaching to at the time. When I first met Feldenkrais in 1976, there would not have been a person in our Feldenkrais training class who would not have known of G. I. Gurdjieff, F. M. Alexander, or Jean Houston, all individuals who were important to Feldenkrais. When I mention these same people today to my Feldenkrais students, or bring up other individuals from my era who were pivotal for me, most of the students have never heard of them.

This disorienting experience, of having the cultural greats of your era nearly disappear for the next generation, hearkens back to a time in 1983 when I went to Israel to study with Feldenkrais. At the time he had just

---

*There are hints that there may be others, but after a thorough search we have not been able to find anything more.

recovered from a stroke and was working a part-time schedule, seeing two or three individuals each day for *Functional Integration* (individual hands-on teaching sessions). He was also working on writing his autobiography. He would write by hand and later I would type what he had written. Many of the names he mentioned were unfamiliar to me, and often I had to go to him for clarification. He was amazed that I was not familiar with many of the historical figures he mentioned. At the time I was in my mid-twenties, and more than fifty years—and a lot of life history—separated us. Nonetheless, he seemed disturbed by this gap in my knowledge. In the afternoons, other students of the Method would come and Feldenkrais would hold court, sitting at a table in front of his wall of books. I remember him best there, reaching for a book on his shelf to make a point, talking on the phone in four languages, arguing with pleasure against whatever position I became too attached to, all the time moving, even when apparently sitting still. . . . Having become intrigued by my historical gaps, he quizzed some of the other students about the same figures from his past and realized that I was not the only one unfamiliar with them. After that he grudgingly began to work with me to add a bit more context for some of the historical figures he mentioned in his autobiography.*

Time moves on and one generation's giant can be the next one's footnote. In editing this volume I experienced a sense of *déjà vu* as I seemed to continue a process started with Feldenkrais so long ago in Tel Aviv, and at the same moment feeling time's footsteps on my back, as some of the greats of my own youth now need to be footnoted as well.

Embodied Wisdom: The Collected Papers of Moshe Feldenkrais contains Feldenkrais's most concise descriptions of the *Feldenkrais Method*. The first two articles—"Bodily Expressions" and "Mind and Body"—are especially complete, lucidly covering many aspects of *Feldenkrais* theory and interspersed with small exercises to embody the ideas. In "Bodily Expressions" he develops at length his thoughts about self-image, a central tenet of his work. The article also includes the most in-depth discussion of the concept

---

*Unfortunately, this autobiography was still in a very rough form when Feldenkrais died and so it was never published.

of reversibility, as it applies to movement, to be found anywhere in his writing. In "Mind and Body" he lays out his arguments for the integrity of body and mind and goes on to talk specifically about his work in this context. All the articles return to the theme of learning, and how the human ability to learn is both our biggest challenge and our greatest hope. Learning is the main theme of Will Schutz's interview, "Movement and the Mind" as well as the transcribed talk "Man and the World." The two articles approach the theme of learning from different angles, but both explore the impressive ability of the human nervous system to adapt and learn. The article "On the Primacy of Hearing," on the other hand, delves into one aspect of the learning process, investigating the relationship of hearing to the development of spatial orientation.

One of the shortest pieces in the book is "On Health," a lovely piece discussing Feldenkrais's ideas about what it means to be healthy in the largest sense. These themes are picked up again in more detail in "Self-Fulfillment Through Organic Learning," a rambling talk artfully edited by Mark Reese. The importance of awareness and its definition is another big theme returning throughout this volume. We can see Feldenkrais developing his early ideas about awareness and learning in the discussion with Aharon Katzir, skillfully edited by Carl Ginsburg. These themes are later forefront in an interview with Edward Rosenfeld from 1973: "The Forebrain: Sleep, Consciousness, Awareness, and Learning."

While Feldenkrais's passion for his work is apparent throughout the book, for the reader with no experience of the *Feldenkrais Method*, it may be challenging to construct from the articles just what the practice of the Method looks like. For this reason, photos of Feldenkrais working have been added to the text. In addition, the first article specifically suggests movement experiments for the reader to help embody the ideas being discussed. I highly recommend taking the time to engage in the proposed experiments, as these early experiences will continue to be helpful throughout the rest of the book. Two articles that discuss the practice of the Method more specifically are "Awareness Through Movement," and "An Interview with Moshe Feldenkrais, *The New Sun*." The first is a version of a handout Feldenkrais used at his institute in Tel Aviv to orient new students to his Method. *The*

Sun interview happened just after the interviewers witnessed a hands-on session. Many of the questions thus focus on Feldenkrais's thinking process as he engages in a session of *Functional Integration.*

Two of the interviews concern the relevance of Feldenkrais's ideas to theater. Richard Schechner, a well-known director, interviews Feldenkrais in "Image, Movement and Actor: Restoration of Potentiality," which includes discussions of self-image, neutrality, and reversibility as applied to acting. When I contacted Schechner in the process of preparing the book, he sent a delightful reminiscence from the time he met Feldenkrais. It is now included at the end of his piece. The interview done by theater professor Joanna Rotté, "Feldenkrais Revisited: Tension, Talent, and the Legacy of Childhood," takes a different, and equally interesting, turn focusing on talent and its development, among other themes.

"The Extraordinary Story of How Moshe Feldenkrais Came to Study Judo," the interview with Dennis Leri, is perhaps the interview where Feldenkrais's personality and style shine through the most clearly. Leri knew Feldenkrais well and gave him the space to expand his story. The result is the weaving of a great tale and a window into Feldenkrais in a relaxed and conversational setting.

Taken together, the articles and interviews become greater than the sum of their parts, forming a diverse and textured whole. The text offers many different points of entry for those unfamiliar with Feldenkrais's ideas and at the same time provides plenty of territory for in-depth study for the serious student of Feldenkrais's work.

This project involved the help and support of many people who generously contributed their expertise and time. I would especially like to thank David Zemach-Bersin, whose knowledge of specific details of Feldenkrais's life and work has proved invaluable in the book's creation and who accompanied me through the project. Dennis Leri has also been extremely helpful in providing steady support and input on a wide range of issues. Lea Wolgensinger has been very generous in providing many of her father's wonderful photos, which have greatly enriched the book.

I would like to remember Michél Silice Feldenkrais, who supported this project in its early stages, before his tragic and untimely death. I would also like to acknowledge his widow Zipora Mandel Silice for her gracious participation. Additional thanks are due to the International Feldenkrais Federation (IFF) for granting permission to include photographs taken by Bob Knighton.

I am grateful to the following people for various kinds of help and advice along the way: Arlyn Zones, Miriam Pfeffer, Eleanor Criswell, Carl Ginsburg, Carol Kress, Kaethe Zemach-Bersin, Donna Ray, Cathie Krieger, Bruce Silvey, Joanna Rotté, Sasha du Lac, and Falk Fedderson.

I would also like to thank Deirdre O'Shea for all her skillful editorial help and Hisae Matsuda for her patience and insight as the project Editor at North Atlantic Books. Finally, I must thank my husband Rafael Núñez, and my daughter Aliana Núñez-Beringer, for creating our cozy world to come home to when the day's work is done.

ELIZABETH BERINGER
San Diego, California
May 2010

PART 1

Articles

1

Bodily Expressions

Translated from the French by Thomas Hanna

"Aspects d'une technique: l'expression corporelle" was written in 1964 and published as a fifteen-page monograph by Éditions Chiron, the publisher of all of Dr. Feldenkrais's French-lanuage books. In 1988, Thomas Hanna, the editor of *Somatics* magazine, translated it into English and published it as "Bodily Expressions," split over two consecutive issues of the magazine. Presented here in one piece, it is one of the earliest writings in the collection and also the most in-depth explanation of Feldenkrais's work available in the shorter article format. As in the original *Somatics* article, we have been able to include photographs taken by Michael Wolgensinger,[1] an accomplished Swiss photographer. Michael Wolgensinger and his wife Luzzi were close friends of Feldenkrais for nearly forty years.—*Ed.*

THE BEHAVIOR OF HUMAN BEINGS IS FIRMLY BASED on the self-image they have made for themselves. Accordingly, if one wishes to change one's behavior, it will be necessary to change this image.

What is a self-image? I would argue that it is a body image; namely, it is the shape and relationship of the bodily parts, which means the spatial and temporal relationships, as well as the kinesthetic feelings. Included with this are feelings and emotions and one's thoughts. All of these form an integrated whole.

How does a self-image come about? Everyone feels that his way of walking, speaking, and behaving is uniquely his own and unchangeable. He totally identifies with this behavior—as if he were born with it. The way he sees objects in space, the way he tracks movements, the way he inclines his head, and the way he looks at things seem to be innate; and he believes it impossible to change any of these things—other than perhaps their rate of speed or intensity or duration.

Despite this belief, everything central to human behavior is acquired only by a long period of learning: to walk, to speak, to see a photo or painting in three dimensions—one's very movements, attitude, and language are acquired purely according to the accidental circumstances of one's place of birth and environment.

Thus, when we learn to speak a second language, we always speak it with an accent—an earlier learning always stands in the way of a new learning. It is always difficult to sit as the Japanese or Hindus do, because earlier habits stand in the way. Thus, whatever the accident of one's birth, the difficulty we experience when attempting to change mental or physical habits has little to do with heredity and everything to do with the general problem of changing any habit that has already been acquired.

It is obvious that the difficulty is not in the habit per se but with the earlier point in time at which these accidental habits were formed. And so it appears that our self-image is acquired purely by accident. Hence, the question arises as to whether it might be possible that one can freely choose new habit patterns which are more appropriate and fitting to one's unique person.

Understand that what is in question here is not simply the replacement of one mode of acting with another, which would be purely a static change. What I am suggesting is a change in our way of acting which aims at a dynamic change in the whole process of one's action. Before we go any further, it may be worthwhile to engage in a brief experiment that will allow one to feel this possibility rather than merely to understand it.

If you lie down on your stomach and bend the right knee so that the lower leg points up towards the ceiling, you will find that the relation of the foot with respect to the leg is highly variable with different people. Everyone does not hold his foot in the same position. This becomes obvious if we place a book on the sole of the foot: The plane of the book will most likely not be parallel with the ceiling, but it will have a particular slant that varies with each individual. One can see that the muscular contractions of the leg and the foot have a particular relationship with one another. Even if the

4

musculature is not supporting a weight, it still will not be in a neutral pattern. The musculature is following a pattern dictated by one's self-image. This uniquely individual pattern is felt subjectively to be both obvious and inevitable. This is because habitual patterns are imprinted in the nervous system. The nervous system reacts to exterior stimulation with this habitual ready-made pattern, for it has no other available pattern of response. In order to bring about the kind of dynamic change we are suggesting, these compulsive patterns need to be removed from the nervous system, leaving it free to act or react—not according to habit, but according to the given external situation.

To change the dynamics of this foot-leg relationship, one need only make about twenty extremely slow movements, with attention fixed upon both the trajectory of the foot and the different parts of the foot. For example, flex and extend the foot with your attention on the movement of the heel. Try to follow this movement and, at the same time, be aware of the movements of the big toe—and, one by one, of each of the other toes. This should be done in the gentlest of ways, reducing the intensity of the movement so as to facilitate the change that will gradually occur.

As you focus on each one of the toes moving in space you will experience very individual differences in the degree of difficulty you will have in perceiving these parts of the foot. The difficulty comes from the fact that these varying degrees of clarity create a discontinuity in the flow of images we have of these bodily parts.

Try another movement pattern with the foot: Move the point of the foot around in a circle while trying to sense the corresponding movement of your heel. If you make a sudden stop, notice how surprisingly difficult it is to know exactly where the heel is in some positions, whereas in other positions it is relatively easy.

Now do the movement of the foot extremely slowly, this time making small arcs rather than a complete circle. Stop at various points of the arc and, again, try to sense the exact position of the point of the foot and the heel in relation to the line of the leg lying on the floor.

Now try to move the point of the foot directly to the left and right while trying to keep track of the opposite movement of the heel. You will notice that the heel does not follow a horizontal line and that it does something quite different at the extreme right and left of its trajectory.

Try another movement pattern: Turn the point of the foot to the inside, which moves the heel outward to the right; then turn the point of the foot back to the outside, but do so by making a small semicircle, sometimes arcing above and sometimes arcing below. Do this movement with extreme slowness until you can turn it into a complete circle of the heel, all the while being aware of the corresponding movement of the point of the foot. Make your tracking of the point of the foot even more precise by thinking, in turn, of the big toe, the second toe, the third toe, the fourth toe, and the little toe. From time to time, reverse the circle and continue until the spatial patterns become easy, simple, and clear—this is to say, until the spatial patterns become just like the usual movements which are a part of our self-image and have the same simplicity, clarity, and easiness.

Do these movements without any extra effort or any attempt to make them difficult. If you become confused, simply stop and start all over again.

One thing you will notice is that each time you find a difficult spot to track there will be a simultaneous change in your breathing. At any moment of confusion, stop and wait until your breathing gradually becomes normal again. After a while, you will notice that the more your breathing remains continuous, the more you will find that the flow of spatial images of heel and toe becomes easier. And you will be surprised how quickly the time then begins to pass.

If you now stretch out the right leg, you will notice that it seems longer. You will experience a change in the kinesthetic sensations not only of the muscles and joints of the right foot but also of the entire right side of your body: The right eye will seem more open—and it actually is. All of the right side of the face will actually be longer and the muscles more relaxed.

If you stand up, you will also notice definite changes in the movement of the right foot and the way it feels against the floor. In fact, there will be various changes noticeable in all of the right side of the body. For example, the head will turn more easily to the right than to the left, and it will go farther to the right. If you lift the right arm slowly upward above your head, bring it back down, and then do the same with the left arm, it is likely you will feel that the right arm is lighter.

Using the same procedure, you can do the same exercise series with the head instead of the heel: Tilt the head, then bring it back up while paying attention to the spatial orientation of the head to different segments of the left side of the body—for example, with the shoulder, the collar bone, the spine, and so forth. You will notice a similar change—a change in the muscular tonus of the entire left side right down to your toes.

In light of all this, certain important conclusions suggest themselves:

1. Even though both sides of the body participated equally in the movements of tilting and righting the head, it was the side subjected to conscious scrutiny that showed changes in muscular tonus, ease of movement, and a greater feeling of well-being. This means that movement, by itself, is of small significance beyond certain improvements in circulation and other minor bodily benefits. Hence, the change occurring in two identically moving sides came from paying conscious attention to one side and becoming clear about its spatial orientation. It is significant that the change takes place only in the side on which one has focused—a fact which indicates that the change has occurred through extrapyramidal pathways of the nervous system.

2. Accordingly, we must conclude that the change took place in the central nervous system itself, inasmuch as the change affected the entire side upon which we had focused.

3. Finally, this change will not immediately pass away but may last from several hours to several days. It depends directly on the amount of time spent in doing the exercise and upon the clarity with which the spatial relations were envisioned.

The significance of what this technique causes to happen in the central nervous system is underlined by the fact that one can obtain the same changes on the opposite side of the body by purely mental effort: namely, by directing one's attention methodically back and forth to the kinesthetic sensa-

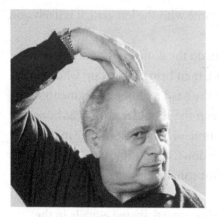

Feldenkrais in the late 1960s.

tions of one side, then another—without any movement whatsoever. Whereas more than half an hour was required to achieve the initial changes on the first side, the other side will show these same changes within a few minutes merely by means of a systematic, point-by-point, conscious survey of the differences between the two sides from top to bottom.

After such a procedure, perhaps the most important thing to emphasize is how satisfying it is to change one's habitual ways of using the head or feet. This change makes one realize how far one's usual habits of self-control are from what they could be—from what they were truly intended to be. This is something we shall attempt to make clear in what follows.

It is evident that there are certain areas of the self-image upon which this exercise in conscious attention has special effectiveness. This is to say that there is a system of priorities which can make such exercises easier and more methodical.

In support of this, an initial observation to be made is that a neonatal human's first relationship with the exterior world is established by means of the mouth. From the beginning, the use of the mouth requires special ways of orienting the head in space. Little by little, the development of our teleceptive senses (hearing, seeing, smelling) requires special movements of the head.

The teleceptive senses, being in pairs that are evenly separated from one another, can correctly judge direction and distance of objects only by head movements. The senses of hearing, seeing, and smelling have a complex neurological function that necessitates head rotation so that the balanced stimulation of the twin sense organs can point the face directly at the source of this stimulation. The head serves as a kind of periscope of the central nervous system in order to bring sensory information into the brain.

In final analysis, the only part of our being that holds a relationship with the external world is the nervous system—the senses and the rest of the body serve only as a means for action and information gathering. It is obvious that the head, bearer of the teleceptive senses, has active participation in all of our relations with external reality. Thus, the way in which the head moves constitutes the essential ingredient in our self-image, and the vertebral column lying below it has an equally important role, because it makes rotation possible in the cervical and lumbar spine.

These considerations show the importance of the skeleton's role in our self-image. The head, resting on the pelvic structure by means of the vertebral column, is involved in every action—passive, active, or orienting—that relates us to the external world.

The thoracic cavity and its respiratory functions are suspended from the vertebrae and are affected by its movements. In return, its movements cannot help but be affected by the respiratory functions. For this reason, the thoracic cavity must not do anything that disturbs the position of the head; instead, it must cooperate in facilitating [the head's] constant orientations. With this in mind, let us look briefly at how this relates to one's self-image.

If, while lying on your back, you do a careful mental survey of your entire body, you will notice that some parts of your body are more easily sensed than others. The parts that are less easily sensed are not part of our conscious actions. Moreover, you will find that during each separate action other bodily areas will be absent from consciousness—indeed, some areas are almost never present in our self-image.

A complete self-image is an ideal rarely attained—namely, an equal awareness of the whole body, every part having the same importance (front, back, and both sides). Everyone has to face the fact that his degree of self-control directly mirrors his self-image. This image is, unfortunately, much more limited than the ideal.

We should recognize as well that the relationship of all sections of our bodies changes in accordance with the different things we do and the different postures we assume. If, for example, you close your eyes and try to hold your index fingers exactly as wide apart as your mouth, you may be astonished to find that you have either overestimated or underestimated the width by as much as three hundred percent.

Or, again, close your eyes and, with the hands, try to indicate the thickness of your chest, front to back. Then try to determine the measurement of the vertical dimensions of your chest in the same way. You will be surprised to discover that your judgment changes each time the position of your hand changes. The three attempts to measure the spatiality of your bodily parts will have resulted in three disparate measurements which are grossly disproportionate.

Here is another experiment you might try: Close your eyes and hold your hands comfortably in front of your face, pointing the right finger directly at your left eye and your left finger at your right eye. Now imagine these lines as rigid rays of light crossing somewhere at the midpoint. Fix that midpoint in space and then take your right thumb and index finger to take hold of that midpoint. Open your eyes and see how far you are off center—if at all.

Then repeat the same thing, this time bringing the left thumb and index finger to the crossover point, and open the eyes again. This is a good way to discover how visual manual errors have a kinesthetic origin.

If one does a detailed examination of persons in this manner and if there are truly gross differences between their self-image and their objective performances, one can be sure that there will be truly gross defects in their control of those sections of their body. For example, people who habitually hold their chest with an exaggerated tightness, as if they had just exhaled, discover that their self-image of the chest is two to three times deeper than the chest actually is. Inversely, people who habitually have an exaggeratedly expanded, inspiratory chest position will underestimate the depth of their chest. A detailed examination of all the body parts yields many such surprises, particularly in the pelvis and the anal-genital region.

Once we come to see that one's degree of self-control directly mirrors one's self-image, we can understand why we find it so difficult to improve our bodily performance by focusing only on the learning of specific actions. Instead, we might well surmise that to improve one's self-image so that it more nearly approximates reality will result in a general improvement in one's bodily actions. And the results of such an improvement would be both quicker and more extensive than the results from any system of exercises that applies only to specific actions.

Muscular Action

It is the musculature, both smooth and striated muscles, that gives us meaningful and comprehensive information about events in the nervous system. Without muscular action, neurological events would show themselves as little more than slow chemical reactions and types of electrical impulses that bear no information of human significance.

If we had only these reactions and impulses as information, we would never know if the nervous system is responding to beauty, if it is experiencing green or red, good or bad, pleasant or unpleasant. Only muscular expression can tell us that. The smooth muscles express the impulses of our internal life, and the striated muscles link up the nervous system with the whole process. As far as we presently know, the muscles are the only means for giving humanly meaningful expression to the chemical and electrical processes of the nervous system.

It is hence of primal importance that the muscular system be thoroughly studied in regard to its relationship with neurological functions. From the outset, we should be clear on this point: Until it reaches the peripheral musculature, no neurological event can be perceived either as a sensation or a feeling, or as a mood or action. And by "periphery," we mean to include the mucous orifices of mouth and anus as well as the musculature of the capillaries and the entire circulatory system.

In itself, the brain appears to be insensible of the majority of excitations which, in the periphery, can cause such lively reactions. In fact, one can become aware of a harmful event in the brain itself only when it causes an action in the periphery—only then does it become conscious.

X-rays or high-frequency waves can burn or destroy bones and internal tissue without being noticed. One becomes conscious of it only when it affects the periphery. Kidney stones and gallstones may form imperceptibly, but they are sharply perceived at the moment they begin dilating the sphincter. We do not feel the destructive process of tooth decay until it begins to affect the capillaries and the gums.

From the beginning to the present, terrestrial life has had to evolve nervous and muscular systems that could adapt with the earthly field of gravitation. Outside of controlling temperature and chemical homeostasis of the body, the nervous and muscular systems are primarily engaged in survival activities, all of which involve locomotion in the field of gravity.

Even our classification of the animal kingdom is based on the animal's mode of locomotion: Fish swim, birds fly, other animals slither, creep, climb, or walk on four legs, or two legs, and so forth.

There is a central feature of all muscular activity that we must bear in mind: If we attempt consecutively to do an easy movement of the finger, then the hand, then the forearm, then the whole arm, trying to judge the relative effort involved in each of these movements, it will be noticed that all of these movements are performed with the same ease. Even so, by simple calculation of work done over gravity, we can determine the foot-pounds of work required for a movement; for example, only so many foot-pounds of work are required for the finger, more foot-pounds for the hand, even more foot-pounds for the forearm, and much, much more work for the entire arm. What this means is that the feeling of muscular effort is not measuring work done, but something else. This "something else" is how the movement is organized: its quality.

The quantity of work done can vary from one foot-pound to a million, while the feeling of effort remains exactly the same. The feeling of increased effort will occur only when there is some type of resistance or disturbance that causes us to mobilize an inappropriately greater effort in order to overcome it. And this feeling of increased effort is obviously not due to an increased amount of work done. Thus, we can conclude, in general, that sensations and feelings tell something about internal organization and about the quality of the mobilization, but not about differences measurable or verifiable as objective realities.

Inasmuch as feelings and sensations do not tell us what is actually taking place, we have no recourse but to avail ourselves of mental processes, of judgment, understanding, and knowledge, if we wish to be certain that what we feel and sense is really what we want to happen. Without such means being called into service, the errors that might occur could very well be fatal.

Our actions are organized according to a self-image that was formed, as it were, by accident. It is a self-image which is made up of feelings and sensations. This being the case, it is elementary to point out that our actions—when based on areas of our self-image that are less than clear—may result in errors, such as doing the opposite of what one thinks one is doing or doing something that has no clear relation with what one feels one is doing. And these actions will occur without any perception of their occurrence.

Earlier, while you were doing the experiment of rotating the heel and toes, it is likely you experienced moments when you were doing movements quite different from what you felt you were doing. As soon as you begin to notice such a mistake, it will cause an abrupt interruption in the flow of spatial images. Rarely does anyone so lose track of his heel or toe to the extent that he no longer knows where the toe and heel are in space or what is being done with either one. This is because we rarely make it a matter of conscious attention to see if there is a direct correspondence between our actions and what we intend.

Usually, we do little more than move according to the self-image that was formed in us from birth up to about fourteen years of age. This vague image usually works more or less satisfactorily, for we rarely need to have a more complete image.

Even though in later life we are capable of much more complex actions, we normally continue making use of the image patterns established during our youth. The time that we have for developing this image is much more continuous then, for it is rarely broken up into occasional learning periods, as is the case for the adult. It is worthwhile noting that this adult discontinuity in subjective learning is a hindrance to higher possibilities of human creativity. This is the question: Are there actions that are so much outside of the self-image of any individual that we do the very opposite of what we had intended when we try to do them?

Here is a movement which will show what I mean: Place the palm of your right hand over the navel, the fingers pointing to the left. Without moving the hand, rotate the elbow around so that it is directly in front of you at a right angle between the forearm and the back of the hand. You may find that you are unable to accomplish this simple movement. If this is the case, place the hand instead on a table and notice how easily you can make a right angle between the back of the hand and the forearm. Then try the earlier movement in a different manner: Keep this right angle between the back of the hand and the forearm and place the palm of the hand on the navel, as you did before. Notice that you can now do it. How is it possible for your hand to do now what it could not do only a moment before? Why was it doing just the opposite of what you wanted it to do? Inasmuch as the hand is the most adroit and frequently used part of our body for making voluntary movements, how is it possible that it cannot obey us? How can the hand so disobey us that the flexor muscles are activated when we actually wish to contract the extensor muscles?

Learning how to execute this movement correctly and in exactly the way we intended takes only a moment. But, as we remarked earlier, it is not simply a question of replacing one action with another, for we are primarily interested in the more dynamic question of how we control ourselves.

To complete and clarify one's self-image by paying attention to the spatial and temporal orientation of one's body can bring about a growth in self-knowledge. The concern to do this is not as unusual as might first be supposed. Creative artists—whether painters, musicians, poets, scientists, or philosophers—attempt to enlarge and clarify their self-image in the particular area of their specialty. For example, a painter before his canvas attempts to take into account his feelings about the image before him, as well as the position and weight of the hand, in order to direct the brush with exactly the precision he feels is necessary. Often the painter will retouch the surface over and over until he achieves the image that meets his satisfaction.

A poet measures not only the meaning of his words but also their length, sounds, and interrelations until their grouping precisely translates his feelings and thoughts. He is doing with words exactly the same thing we were doing with our heel a moment ago. He, as well, widens and clarifies what he is doing, thus making his self-image more precise and more aware in this particular domain.

In the foregoing examples of the painter, the poet, and the movements of the foot, a simple mechanical repetition would result in no more than a static change; it would not result in any kind of developmental process. This raises the question: What is the essential quality of a human practice which makes for a broadening and clarification of one's self-image? Obviously, there must somehow or other be a progression in one's self-awareness that brings about either new or better actions, just as the practice with the heel leads to better usage of the entire leg and its component parts. Without conscious attention to what one is feeling during an action and without applying this attention directly to the entire movement resulting from these actions, no development will occur—simple mechanical repetition will never make this come about.

Thus, the postman, despite his daily repeated journeys, will never become a long-distance sprinter until he turns his attention to his movements and becomes conscious of the spatial and temporal orientation of his self-image. Likewise, an athlete who contents himself with mechanical repetition will achieve the most minimal progress.

If there is to be a progressive development of one's self-image, it is necessary to focus on completing the image in all of its dimensions—not simply in those dimensions with which one is most familiar. One does not know how breathing might be improved by an improvement in the functions of our digestion, nor what repercussion these two dimensions might have on our vision or our memory. A mathematician who is also a musician is not like other musicians; nor is the poet-musician like other poets—the added dimensions change the whole. It is when a self-image becomes more or less complete that we have a Leonardo da Vinci or a William Shakespeare.

With these things in mind, let us see if we can gain a better understanding of muscular activity. The first thing to note is that the same muscle can respond to very different stimuli: The muscle of the eyelid can, for example, make a clonic movement during certain states of fatigue or make a reflex contraction when an insect flies into the eye or contract when one has the voluntary intention to close the eye. In each case, the quality of the muscular contraction is different.

All voluntary movements, for instance, have one thing in common: They are reversible; i.e., at any time in the trajectory of the movement one can stop and go in the reverse direction, or do something altogether different. In those parts of one's self-image where a complete learning has not yet occurred, this kind of reversibility is not possible. If, for example, one attempts to turn the head to the right while simultaneously trying to turn the eyes to the left, one instantly feels what it is like for a movement to be nonreversible. If one attempts to make these two movements twenty times, all the while paying attention to the rhythm of one's breathing—and continues doing this until it becomes as simple as moving the eyes in the same direction—one will discover that there is a change in the muscular tonus at the back of the neck on the side of the head's rotation. If the head is turned to the left and then to the right, one discovers that the right side is freer and that the degree of rotation is clearly greater to the right than to the left. Moreover, the rotation to the right is easier and more fluid. The right side now has the factor of reversibility, as well as a wider angle of turning.

There is a distinct advantage in achieving reversibility: Not only does the movement become more fluid, but it also has a greater range of adaptability. In our everyday lives, we tend to turn our head and eyes together simultaneously, and this becomes habitual. The reverse movement—turning the eyes opposite from the head—is so rare that some persons have never done it.

The movements of the torso and arms have the same habitual parallelism as the head and eyes. Because of this habit, one does not have the skill of reversibility when one attempts to move the arms in an opposite direction from the head and eyes. As an example, try this: Place the palm of your right hand behind your head and the palm of the left hand on your forehead and try to rotate the head right and left. Instead of rotating the head, many will rotate the head, eyes, arms, and torso right and left like a single block. Their habitual self-image has taken over, and they are quite unaware of what they are actually doing, even when you point it out to them.

Because these habitual movement patterns assert themselves despite our efforts to do otherwise, they can be considered compulsive. The habitual pattern shoves aside the intended movement pattern, but one does not have the least awareness of what is happening.

When the absence of reversibility is this pronounced, very careful retraining is necessary for the person to become conscious of the difference between what he intends to do and what he actually does. When the skill of reversibility is acquired, the learner has the same feeling that one has in solving a puzzling problem. It is the feeling of having arrived at a greater freedom in one's self-control.

Certain esoteric disciplines make full use of the following technique for training reversibility: The learner suddenly has to freeze in whatever position he happens to be at the instant the teacher commands him—and to keep holding this position, no matter how strange or uncomfortable it may be. But by deliberately holding still until the command to relax, the learner becomes conscious of all the typically habituated and inefficient ways in which his body's parts are arranged. When movement is resumed, the learner has an enhanced consciousness that is the first step in learning reversibility. Gurdjieff[2] calls this the "Stop Technique" and uses it extensively.

By a careful use of methods of this kind one can overcome the bodily limitations caused by an arrested development in one's self-image. The improvement of this self-image carries with it an expansion of the range and number of movement patterns at one's disposal. Thus, improving our skill of reversibility goes hand in hand with a general improvement of our conscious temporal and spatial orientation.

This orientation is so closely bound up with conscious functions that it seems to permeate all conscious activities. We really do not have control of ourselves unless, for example, our eyes and head have their familiar orientation with space and the vertical dimension established by the gravitational field.

If you ever have the experience of awakening in a bed and room unfamiliar to you, you will feel, at the instant of awakening, that you are neither in command of yourself nor your situation. Even when wide awake, you may experience a rupture in the flow of consciousness when there is a sudden surprise or a sudden change in your spatial orientation. For example, if you are ascending a stairway expecting one more step at the top than there actually is, the abrupt surprise is both a mechanical shock to the body and an experiential shock to the flow of consciousness. The same interruption in consciousness also occurs if there is one less step than you expected when descending a stairway.

The return to normal consciousness after such an interruption is accompanied by the question, "Where am I?" Subjectively, the gap in our usual flowing images of spatial orientation is normally experienced as a gap in consciousness.

We can be sure that this relation between consciousness and spatial orientation has important consequences. A methodical and careful application of the concept of reversibility to one's self-image has, over time, the following results:

1. It makes us conscious of the shapes and interrelationships of the skeleton.
2. It both reduces and equalizes the prevailing muscular tonus.
3. It reduces the amount of effort expended in all we do.
4. It simplifies the way in which we mobilize ourselves for any particular action.
5. It enhances our sensitivity, allowing us to take notice of even small aberrations from the norm.
6. It improves our ability to orient ourselves spatially.
7. It adds versatility to the way our intelligence functions.
8. It reduces fatigue, thus increasing our capacity for work and endurance.
9. It improves posture and breathing, thereby rejuvenating the body.
10. It improves one's health and capacity for action.
11. It improves coordination in all that we do.
12. It makes all learning easier, mental or physical.
13. It leads to a deeper self-awareness.

When the muscular tonus is reduced while being accompanied by an enhanced skeletal awareness, the skeletal structure is able to fulfill its function of nullifying the vertical component of gravity. This frees the musculature from any weight-bearing function, so that our intentional actions are performed with the least possible effort, ideally with an almost zero effort.

In effect, this means, for example, that if one stands with the legs too far apart, movements from left to right are more effortful than would be the case if the legs were closer together. By the same token, this wide-apart stance means that forward and backward movements are possible only by first aligning the skeleton with the vertical forces of gravity; once the vertical compression of gravity is nullified, one can move forward or backward with minimal effort. Theoretically, the only effort required in moving should be expended in overcoming the resistance factors of air pressure and of friction.

A general improvement in the way we use our skeleton allows us to enjoy the full range of movements of the joints and intervertebral disks. All too often, the bodily limitations that we believe are due to not being limber are, instead, caused by a habitual contraction and shortening of our muscles of which we are not conscious. Unwittingly, our postures become distorted, and the joints of our bodies suffer unequal pressures.

Degeneration of the joint surfaces imposes, in its turn, a further restriction of muscular activity so as to avoid pain and discomfort in movement. Thus, a vicious circle is established, which gradually distorts the skeleton, the spine, and the intervertebral disks, resulting in an elderly body whose range of movements is reduced long before we have become old. Actually, age has little to do with this sad event. On the contrary, it is quite possible to restore the body's ability to perform every movement of which the skeleton is capable.

Up until sixty years of age, anyone of good health who is not suffering serious illness can attain this optimal ability with little more than an hour of retraining for each year of one's life. It is possible to attain this condition even beyond sixty years—depending on the person's intelligence and will to live.

The Essential Unity of Mind and Body

The central idea behind all we are discussing is the following: The mental and physical components of any action are two different aspects of the same function. The physical and mental components are not two series of

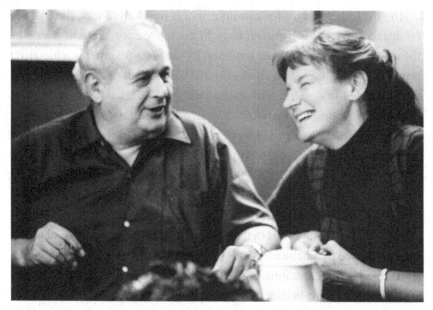

Feldenkrais with Luzzi Wolgensinger, Zurich in the late 1970s.

phenomena, which are somehow linked together; but, rather, they are two aspects of the same thing, like two faces of the same coin. Most likely, the serial, linear nature of language undergirds the serial nature of our thinking and makes the simultaneous expression of these separate aspects possible.

Unless one creates a special vocabulary or a system of notation, such as is used in mathematics, one has little choice other than to keep these two aspects separate—even if one prefers not to do so. Even highly abstract topics, such as number, are not independent of physiological support. The speed of our thinking is closely tied to the speed of our motor cortex functions. The time it takes mentally to count from twenty to thirty is longer than the time it takes to count from one to ten. This is because even nonverbal thinking, such as this, remains caught within the task of articulating numbers, which, in the former instance, takes longer than the simpler numbers of one to ten. By the same token, if we think "to the right" or "to the left," it will immediately activate the muscles of the eye.

With training, the human nervous system can learn to eliminate these muscular activities of the larynx and the eye, thereby speeding up the mental

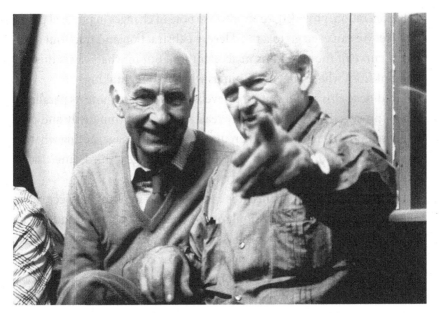

Feldenkrais with the photographer Michael Wolgensinger, 1981.

process. Even so, our thinking remains limited to the speed at which the motor cortex can function. The simple act of reading this page is limited by the speed of visual perception. But even in this instance, we can accelerate our mental processes by disassociating them from the muscular processes that usually accompany the act of reading.

What is important is that thinking involves a physical function which supports the mental process. No matter how closely we look, it is difficult to find a mental act that can take place without the support of some physical function. Contemporary thinking about the structure of matter indicates that it is only a manifestation of energy—something more attenuated, such as thinking itself.

It is our familiarity with certain phenomena that makes it difficult to appreciate them clearly. For us, speed is a very real thing—tangible and measurable. Even so, we can neither touch nor measure speed. It is an abstraction. In order to measure speed, we have to take note of changes in certain physical points in space. But we can go further by measuring an abstraction of the already abstract idea of speed: that is, we can measure acceleration and deceleration, provided we always take note of changes in physical points in space. We can even go to a third level of abstraction and trace out a statistical curve of the variations in acceleration. But in what way is this any different from what happens within us when we are thinking?

Holding to this analogy of three levels of abstraction, note its parallel to mental process: For example, I may read a page absentmindedly and then ask myself if I understand it. Whereupon I reread the page, noting whether or not I am comprehending it. Then I read the page a third time, asking myself why I did not understand it the first time.

In a brief essay such as this, it is impossible to treat this subject rigorously. Even so, we can see the similarity of these two analogies, and we can appreciate that a change in speed is possible only with an accompanying change in the physical process supporting it. Any change in the latter means a change in the former. Mental process produces a change in its physical substratum, and a change in the physical substratum of thinking manifests itself as a mental change. In both instances, looking for the origin of the change is futile: Neither a change in speed nor a change in thought is possible without a change in its physical substratum.

The state of wakeful consciousness is made up of four elements: movements, sensations, feelings, and thoughts. If these four activities are absent, one soon falls asleep. It is taken as a matter of fact that movement and sensation are central nervous system functions; but, beyond this, we are proposing that mental process is the same kind of function. And we shall attempt to show that feelings are also functions of the central nervous system.

The reaction of fear involves a violent contraction of the flexor muscles—especially the abdominals—and breathholding. This is accompanied by a series of vasomotor disturbances: the pulse quickens, perspiration increases, and, in extreme cases, trembling and defecation may occur. Many a soldier has experienced this at the moment of quitting the trenches for the first bayonet charge. The strong flexor contraction is accompanied by a simultaneous inhibition of its antagonist, the extensor muscles, causing the knees to bend and making it difficult to stand upright.

A neonatal infant has very little sensitivity to external stimuli: it has only a slight reaction to light, sound, odor, or even to moderate pinching. But if that infant feels a sudden drop, a violent contraction takes place in the flexor muscles: breathing stops, crying ensues, the pulse quickens, and vasomotor disturbances occur. There is a striking similarity between a just-born baby's reaction to falling and an adult's reaction to the fear of falling.

Because the reaction to falling is present at birth, it is innate—independent of learned experience. The lowering of the head, the folding inward, the knee flexion, the trembling, and the lack of extensor tonus characteristic of a person in the throes of anxiety or fear—these are all part of the general contraction of the flexor muscles.

A few weeks later, when the baby's hearing is more acute, the same kind of violent reaction happens with a sudden loud noise. In all sections of the nervous system where myelinization is not yet completed, there is a diffusion of excitation to adjacent nerves and branches of nerves. The eighth cranial nerve has two branches, the cochlear and the vestibular, and the latter branch innervates the semicircular canals. A sudden loss in support of the neonate causes an intense excitation of the vestibular branch due to the reaction of the semicircular canals to the fall. When the cochlea reacts to a loud noise, the excitation of the cochlear branch diffuses over the vestibular branch, creating the same reaction that occurs during a fall.

The reaction pattern that we have found in anxious or fearful adults is produced by stimulation of the vestibular branch of the eighth cranial nerve. The disturbances that are typical of anxiety—vertigo, vomiting, and other symptoms—are the same as those generally seen when the vestibular functions are disturbed.

Thus, we have established what is the underlying pattern in the formation of anxiety complexes, ingrained states of fear, indecisiveness, and chronic self-doubt. Additionally, we have pointed out the interdependence of feelings on the one hand and central nervous system functions on the other hand, showing how they affect bodily posture and create typical patterns of muscular tonus. And we have done this by focusing closely on a few of the many examples of these phenomena.

In summing up, we would like to reiterate how crucial the control of musculature is in the control of self. Careful examination of habitual posture, and the patterns of muscular contraction causing it, make it possible to infer which areas of the motor cortex are subject to ongoing abnormal excitation and which areas are subject to ongoing inhibition.

We should bear in mind that life is a fast-moving flow of successive states of the central nervous system and that each state, no matter how complex, represents a gestalt which is indivisible. It is impossible to think both "yes" and "no" at the same instant. No matter how complex any particular idea, act, or experience may be, it represents a whole action of one's whole being.

And if one's whole state of ongoing excitations and inhibitions is such that every thought and action always activates the same regions, we have a good description of the state of obsession. Such states of the nervous system can be smoothed out to normalcy by drugs which act upon the same regions of excitation and inhibition. When similar results sometimes occur in psychotherapy, they are attended by changes in both posture and general muscular tonus.

Let us say once again that the state of the cortex is directly observable on the body's periphery by these configurations of posture and muscular tonus. A change in the central nervous system always means a change in these configurations. Each, as we have pointed out, is the other side of the same coin.

It is obvious that a technique for reducing muscular tonus and methodically improving one's self-image has a significance that can scarcely be overestimated. Such a technique makes it clear that when self-control is defective, something else is defective: there is arrested self-development. Hence, the correction of these defects should not be experienced as the "treatment of an illness," but, rather, as the rekindling of growth and development of one's self.

This technique, developed over the course of two decades, has been elaborated in two directions: One, working directly with the individual by manipulation; and the other, working in a different fashion with fifty persons, or more.

We should not terminate these remarks without a final observation: Considering the organizational levels of the central nervous system (the rhinic, which controls the body's internal milieu; the limbic, which controls the outward expression of inner needs; and the supralimbic, which is

24

still evolving and which allows humans not only to act and speak but to know what we are doing and saying), it is obvious that to become conscious of our body's spatial orientation is to come to know ourselves in depth and in clarity. In this way, we take charge again of our personal evolution, moving in the direction already marked out for us by the whole process of evolution.

2

Mind and Body

In 1959, Gerda Alexander, founder of the system known as "Eutony," organized a historic conference of somatic thinkers in Copenhagen, where her school was located. Gerda Alexander and Moshe Feldenkrais were friends and mutually supportive of each other's work and ideas. Entitled "The Release of Tension and the Re-education of Muscular Movement," the conference included a mix of classes, demonstrations, and lectures. Practitioners in the field of what we would today call Somatics gathered from all over Europe, making the conference a unique event. "Mind and Body" is an article Dr. Feldenkrais developed from a presentation he gave at this conference.

The original publication of "Mind and Body" was in *Systematics: The Journal of The Institute for the Comparative Study of History, Philosophy and the Sciences* in 1964. The Institute was founded by J. G. Bennett, an eclectic spiritual teacher rooted in the lineage of G. I. Gurdjieff and P. D. Ouspensky.[1] Feldenkrais was very interested in their ideas and interacted with many people in the Gurdjieff lineage during his post–World War II years living in London. The journal was founded to create a dialogue with scientists and other thinkers whose interests intersected with Bennett's approach. "Systemics," as Bennett developed the term, referred to autonomous components of a system that interact to form the whole.—*Ed.*

The way the mind and the body are united has preoccupied human beings throughout the centuries. "A healthy mind in a healthy body" and similar sayings show a conception of one kind of unity. In other teachings, the healthy mind makes a healthy body.

I believe that the unity of mind and body is an objective reality. They are not just parts somehow related to each other, but an inseparable whole while functioning. A brain without a body could not think; at least, the continuity of mental functions is assured by corresponding motor functions.

Let me substantiate this point by some examples:

1. It takes us longer to think the numbers from twenty to thirty than from one to ten, although the numerical intervals are the same between one and ten and twenty to thirty. The difference is that the amount of time needed for thinking the numbers is proportional to the time needed to utter them aloud. So one of the "purest" abstractions—counting—is inextricably linked with the muscular activity through its nervous organization.

   In general, in counting objects we find that the motor elements of sight and speech keep down the speed of thought to their own rate of activity. Most people cannot think clearly without mobilizing the motor function of the brain enough to become aware of the word patterns representing the thought. It is of course possible with sufficient training partially to *inhibit* the motor aspect of the thinking and thus increase the facility of thinking.

2. Macular vision—that is, distinct, clear seeing—is limited to a very small area at a time. To perceive clearly the content of what we see while reading takes us the time necessary for the muscles of the eyes to scan the area under inspection. Here again, we see the functional unity of perception and motor function.

These examples indicate that an improvement in speed and clarity of thought may be obtained by reducing the extent of body movement and smoothing the performance of the muscular controls.

Jacobson* asserts that when deep muscular relaxation is obtained, it is difficult, or even impossible, to think without noticing tension in some muscles. Even when picturing an object with closed eyes, one senses a tensioning of the eye muscles.

Also, note how persistently we retain the same thoughts and the same modes of action throughout our lives—for example, how we use the same patterns of the speaking apparatus producing the same voice so that we can be identified by it for decades on end. This is equally true of our handwriting, our carriage, etc.; so long as there is no marked change in these, there is no change in our jokes, attitudes, and moods.

We have no sensation of the inner workings of the central nervous system. We can feel their manifestations only as far as the eye, the vocal apparatus, the facial mobilization, and the rest of the body provoke our awareness. This is the state of consciousness!

There is little doubt in my mind that the motor function, and perhaps the muscles themselves, are part and parcel of our higher functions. This is true not only of those higher functions like singing, painting, and loving, which are impossible without muscular activity, but also of thinking, recalling, remembering, and feeling.

Let us consider feeling in more detail; I may feel joyful, angry, afraid, disgusted. I am buoyant, my breath even, my face at the point of smiling—I feel gay. My motor attitude is quite different when I feel disgusted—then my face is that of a man on the brink of, or immediately after, vomiting. I clench my lower jaw, my fists, my breath is held but pulse accelerated, eyes and head move in jerks, my neck stiff—I am angry and am ready to hurt, but I am trying not to let myself go. I am afraid, I scream, I am trying to get away, or I am frozen stiff.

There is usually a motor pattern sufficiently clear even for an objective evaluation of the intensity of my feeling. Which comes first—the motor pattern or the feeling? The question has been the object of many

---

*Edmund Jacobson (1888–1983) created a progressive relaxation method in the early part of the twentieth century. He is the author of *Progressive Relaxation*, University of Chicago Press, 1938.

famous theories. I stress the view that basically they form a single function. We cannot become conscious of a feeling before it is expressed by a motor mobilization and, therefore, there is no feeling so long as there is no body attitude.

Re-education

There are two major roads for changing a person's behavior—either through the psyche or through the body. However, real change has to be brought about in a way which allows both the body and the psyche to be changed simultaneously. If the approach is not integral but through either the psyche or the body separately, the change will last only as long as the person has not lost the awareness of it, and has not resumed spontaneous habitual patterns. However, by scanning one's own body image, one can detect the return of the unwanted, habitual muscular function some time before it occurs, and can then either inhibit or facilitate it by an act of will.

The advantage of approaching the unity of mental and muscular life through the body lies in the fact that the muscle expression is simpler because it is concrete and easier to locate. It is also incomparably easier to make a person aware of what is happening in the body, and therefore the body approach yields faster and more direct results. On acting on the significant parts of the body, such as the eyes, the neck, the breath, or the pelvis, it is easy to effect striking changes of mood on the spot. I have achieved clear results with a group technique which can also be self-taught.

A few examples may be useful.

Mr. B. was in a mental institution for three years, where he had analysis and later was given electric shock treatment. He left the institution when no further improvement could be reasonably foreseen. When he was re-educated by our method to make only a few more or less normal breathing movements, he dreamt that he was in the bathroom, the walls of which suddenly fell apart, exposing him to onlookers. This dream continued for ten consecutive nights until a complete change in breathing took place. A marked beneficial change in the person's behavior occurred during those days, the forerunner of still further improvement.

Professor Z., who was one of the first psychiatrists to associate himself with my method, has published a remarkable case of a patient in one of his wards, about whom no useful clues were obtained after one hundred sessions of psychotherapy. At the weekly meeting of the medical staff, the somatic approach was suggested. The person was put in an embryo-like position and a certain degree of relaxation and improved breathing brought about. After four sessions a sufficient amount of significant information was obtained, providing a definite course of treatment. This example shows that for purposes of diagnosis, assuming the oneness of mind and body *and* working on the body provide a new outlook which reveals relations between apparently unrelated facts.

Old age, for instance, begins with the self-imposed restriction on forming new body patterns. First, one selects attitudes and postures to fit an assumed dignity and so rejects certain actions, such as sitting on the floor or jumping, which then soon become impossible to perform. The resumption and reintegration of even these simple actions has a marked rejuvenating effect not only on the mechanics of the body but also on the personality as a whole.

Standards of Normality

In my examination of the bodies of several thousand people before and during re-education, I have found there are some norms for the definition of health and normality. In particular I have looked at the distribution of tonus throughout the bodies of these people. Though it is difficult to do full justice to these concepts of health and normality in a few words, the general principles can be drawn.

For example, the head must have no tendency to move in particular directions. The "normal" head should have easy access to all directions of the anatomically possible range of movements. In fact, the factor limiting movements of the body in general should be the skeleton structure and not *muscular* tightness. Actually, every adult uses only a part of the theoretical possibilities of the human frame.

Also, the healthy coordinated movements of the body as a whole obey the mechanical principle of least action, which means the muscles are designed to work in step and perform their tasks with the least expenditure of metabolic energy. In view of these principles governing the operations of the whole human frame, one can decide on normal and abnormal behavior.

To make these norms of normality have universal application, we must view human beings in their entirety. A person is made of three entities: the nervous system, which is the core; the body—skeleton, viscera, and muscles—which is the envelope of the core; and the environment, which is space, gravitation, and society. These three aspects, each with its material support and its activity, together give a working picture of a human being.

There is a functional correspondence between the core (the nervous system) and the outside physical world, or even the social environment. This relationship can be much closer and more vital than even between some adjacent parts of the nervous system itself. Think, for instance, of men going deliberately to face death in order to preserve an established social order. In this case, the ties of a nervous system to a social order may be stronger than those with the body itself, so that some individuals sacrifice the first two parts of themselves to preserve the third. It is to ignore reality, if one intends to make a change in the behavior of a person and disregard, even for a moment, any one of the three constituents of existence.

The nervous system relates itself to the body through the nerves and the hormonal chemistry, and to the outside world through the nerve endings and through the senses, which give information about position in space, pain, touch, and temperature. The nervous system has no *direct* perception of the outside world. What this means is that the distinction between the self and the outside world is a function which must be developed or learned. The system slowly and gradually sorts out the signals of information coming in from the body and from the outside, and recognizes which is which.

The development of this process leads to a clearer and clearer distinction between signals derived from the body (the self) and those derived from the outside world. The former become known as "I" and the latter as "not I." This is the beginning of consciousness; by learning to recognize how our bodies are oriented we come to know ourselves. Subjective and objective realities are thus organically dependent on the motor elements (the nerves, the muscles, and skeleton), which are oriented by and react to the gravitational field.

Gravity is a major aspect of reality and plays an important part in constituting our normality. But we are so accustomed to the gravitational field that we have to *learn* about its existence. The same is true of consciousness, which is continuous so long as the sequence of bodily orientational cues is uninterrupted. How organic this body orientation is to consciousness can only be realized when there is a break in the connection between them. When we wake up to consciousness after fainting or anesthesia, the first thought is "Where am I?" When there is a break in the sequence of orientational cues, as when we fail to find the expected next step, there is a momentary lapse of consciousness. The jolt is so violent that for a moment we lose the ability to direct ourselves.

The term *orientation* is used here in its widest sense, including the distinction between "I" and "not I" in the social field, with all its ramifications. And of course one can see more clearly in the skeleton than anywhere else attitudes of submission, of arrogance, of insignificance, or of importance. An immense field for inquiry is opened once the organic ties of social orientation are followed up into the muscles, nerves, and skeleton. Not only can individual development or abnormality be followed through the body, but so can even wider cultural and racial differences in attitudes.

The introversion, the nonattachment, and the indifference of the Hindu with corresponding looseness of hip joints, and the extroverted, holding-on, time-is-money attitude of the industrial nations (with their utter inability to sit cross-legged), are a few examples. Of course, to soften and bring to normal one's hip joints, one must spend time, look at oneself, give up something, detach oneself from something else.

In human beings a "normal" action can be either unconscious and automatic or fully conscious and aware. Almost all activity which evolved phylogenetically with the human species is common to the entire animal world. This activity becomes more and more complex or aware with the higher members of the tree of evolution. Still, phylogenetically acquired activity is always expressed in abstract terms and is, therefore, unchangeable, as there are no means to affect an abstraction. On the other hand, individually acquired action (ontogenetic action) pertains to the senses. Such action can be altered or learned as one can become aware of actual differences, such as the extent of the effort, its coordination in time, the body sensation, the spatial configuration of the body segments, the standing, the breathing, the wording, etc.

This kind of awared learning is complete when the new mode of action becomes automatic or even unconscious, as all habits do. The advantage of a habit acquired by awareness is that when it shows unfitness or maladjustment when confronted with reality, it easily provokes new awareness and so helps one to make a fresh and more efficient change.

My inmost belief is that, just as anatomy has helped us get an intimate knowledge of the working of the body, and neuroanatomy an understanding of some activities of the psyche, so will understanding of the somatic aspects of consciousness enable us to know ourselves more intimately. Tension is self-destructive. In the future, we should be able to *direct* the forces that generate tension not just to release it, but also in order to improve human functioning.

Techniques for Individual Teaching

In individual teaching I use my hands to produce the desired alignment of the different segments of the body. The effects are very difficult to describe but some sort of idea can be given.

I never deal directly with the affected part or articulation of the body before I bring about an improvement in the head-neck relationship and in breathing. In turn, improvement in the head and neck and in breathing cannot be achieved without correcting the spine and thorax configuration. Again, to do this, the pelvis and abdomen must be corrected. In practice, therefore, the procedure is a successive series of adjustments, each one allowing a further improvement in the segment just dealt with.

Before using this technique, one must experience it oneself first, in order to acquire the necessary delicacy of touch and clear sense of which muscle group or segment needs attention first and which needs it at all.

The peripheral trouble is usually largely dissipated when the spine-head relationship is improved, so that very little work is necessary at the periphery to bring its functioning up to the level of the rest of the body.

I insist on thirty to forty sessions on a daily basis and then two or three sessions a week until the major complaint is gone. Normally, in about fifty percent of the cases, pains and inability to use a body part disappear before the daily sessions are over.

I begin with the person lying on his or her back. This position is meant to reduce most of the influence of gravity on the body, freeing the nervous system. The reaction of the nervous system to the pull of gravity is a habit, and under these circumstances, there is no way to bring the muscles to respond differently to the same stimulus, which is the major means of re-educating the body. Obviously, it is difficult to bring about any real change in the nervous system without reducing or eliminating the effect of gravity.

In due course I reach people by using thirty different body situations, going to sitting, standing, walking, and balancing on two wooden rollers. Some further details of individual work will become clear with the description of the group techniques.

Group Techniques

A group consists of thirty to forty people. They may be people from the age of fifteen to sixty or more. For example, a particular group I have taught consisted of men and women suffering from sciatica, discal hernia, frozen shoulders, and similar complaints. Most of the group were over thirty-five and had been wearing corsets for many years. Other groups may be composed of teachers, actors, singers, dancers, etc.

I begin by asking people to lie on their backs (after the same principle of reducing gravity) and learn to scan themselves. That is, they examine attentively the contact of their bodies with the floor and gradually learn to detect considerable differences—points where the contact is feeble or nonexistent and others where it is full and distinct. This training develops awareness of the location of the muscles producing weak contact through permanent excessive tension, thus holding parts of the body up off the floor. Some improvement in tension reduction can be achieved through muscular

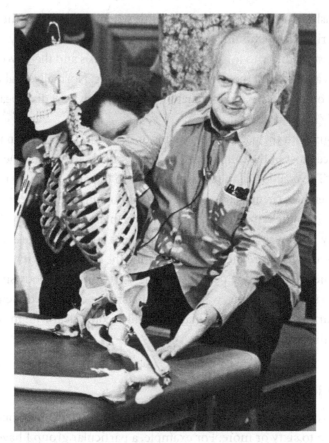

Feldenkrais teaching, 1977.

awareness alone, but beyond that no improvement will be carried over into normal life unless people increase their awareness of the skeleton and its orientation. Here the most difficult joints are the hip joints. Awareness of the location and function of these joints is nonexistent in Western cultures, as compared with that of people who sit on the ground and not on chairs. The chair sitter is almost without exception completely out of place when locating the hip joints. Moreover, chair sitters incorrectly use their legs as if they were articulated at imaginary points in the body image and not where they actually are.

I usually make clear that the point of my work is to lead to awareness in action, or the ability to make contact with one's own skeleton and muscles and with the environment practically simultaneously. This is not "relaxation," for true relaxation can be maintained only when doing nothing. The aim is *not* complete relaxation but healthy, powerful, easy, and pleasurable exertion. The reduction of tension is necessary because efficient movement should be effortless. Inefficiency is sensed as effort and prevents doing more and better.

The gradual reduction of useless effort is necessary in order to increase kinesthetic sensitivity, without which a person cannot become self-regulating. The Weber-Fechner* law shows clearly that this is so. This law states that for a wide range of human sensation and activity, the difference in stimulus that produces the least detectable difference in sensation is always the same ratio to the whole stimulus. For example, if I hold a twenty-pound weight, I cannot detect a fly sitting on it because the least detectable difference of stimulus is from 1:20 to 1:40 and therefore at least half a pound must be added or subtracted from the carried weight to become aware of the change. If I hold a feather, the weight of a fly makes a great difference. Obviously, then, in order to be able to tell differences in exertion one must first reduce the exertion. Finer and finer performance is possible only if the *sensitivity*—that is, the ability to *feel* the difference—is improved. For this reason group work begins with small discoveries in muscle awareness.

Another important feature of the group work is the continued novelty of situation that is maintained throughout the course. Once the novelty wears off, awareness is dulled and no learning takes place. If a configuration needs repetition, I teach it in tens and even hundreds of variations until they are mastered.

---

*Ernst Heinrich Weber (1795–1878) was the first person to study people's ability to perceive sensory contrast in a systematic fashion. Gustav Theodor Fechner (1801–1887) later extended Weber's findings experimentally, theoretically, and mathematically. Their law asserts that the just noticeable difference in any sensation results from a change in the stimulus, which bears a constant ratio to the value of the stimulus. The law applies to sound, light, and numerical cognition as well as kinesthetic sensitivity. The Weber-Fechner law is an essential part of Feldenkrais's explanation of his *Method*. See also pages xvi–xvii, and 101.

All exercises are arranged to produce a neat change in sensation at the end of the lesson and usually a more or less lasting effect. This enables pupils to find connections between different parts of the body, as for instance between the left shoulder blade and right hip joint, or between the eye muscle and the toes.

To produce the mental ease necessary for the reduction of useless efforts, the group is repeatedly encouraged to learn to do a little *less* well than is possible when trying hard to be less fast, less vigorous, less graceful, etc. They are often asked to do the utmost and then deliberately to do a little less. This is more important than it might seem. For if enabled to feel progress while not tensing, pupils have the sensation of being able to do better, which induces more progress. Achievements that otherwise may need numerous hours of work can be obtained in twenty minutes with this attitude of mind and body.

Special mention must be made of very small, barely perceptible movements that I use extensively. They reduce involuntary contraction in the muscles in an astonishing way; in a few minutes by working on one leg or arm, for example, it may be made to feel longer and lighter than the other. After the lesson the pupils keep on feeling what the new way of action is, and the sensation of the light and long member is continuously contrasted by the other, which feels clumsy and awkward in comparison.

Very often one half—the right or left—is worked with during a lesson, and the other half is left as it was. Again, for hours afterwards, pupils carry with them two standards in their bodies—their habitual one, and the proposed better one. They keep feeling the difference until the clumsy side eases up. In this way students learn to ease up, so to speak, from within. This promotes the transfer of learning from the action worked on, to other actions, completely different. The transfer of learning is essentially personal and differs from one individual to the other. One may feel the change in speaking, another person in ways of attending or observing.

Another principle in the group technique is the scanning of the body image, which is done in two parallel ways. One way consists of producing a sensation of length, width, and lightness in one side of the body, by actually moving the body, as explained above. The other half of the body is brought to feel the same sensation by mental scanning *alone*. The mental scanning consists of listening and becoming aware of the difference of sensation in the motor memory of the muscles of the two halves, and the sensation of change of orientation in space.

The other way consists of scanning the body on *both* sides from the start, directing attention to the sensation of the distances between different parts of the body on either side until these sensations correspond to the actual difference.

Another part of the training focuses on improving voluntary movements. In all voluntary acts two phases follow each other so swiftly that it is difficult to note the time delay between one and the other. The preparatory phase is the mobilization of the body attitude needed for the action. The second phase is the performance of the action. Because there is a minute interval of time between these phases it is possible to learn to inhibit or enhance the preparatory mobilization by choice. When there is choice, we can complete the action or else prevent it and cancel the preparatory attitude entirely. In the group, we work on clarifying the delay between the preliminary attitude for action and its completion. This clarification or awareness improves the fluency and voluntary control of movements.

Many exercises use induction, both positive and negative—the aftereffects of prolonged, sustained efforts. For example, stand with your right side close to a wall and press against the wall with the back of your hand as if to push it away. After maintaining this pressure for about a minute, stop. Then leave your right arm free to do as it wishes. It will rise and lift itself to shoulder height with a peculiar lightness like floating. If you voluntarily lower your arm and leave it free again, the same thing will happen several times, but with decreasing intensity. This exercise shows how sustained effort can induce movement after the effort stops.

But whatever the exercise or the principle used, the lesson is so arranged that without concentration, without trying to sense differences, without real attention, pupils cannot proceed to the next stage. Repetition, just mechanical repetition without attention, is discouraged, made impossible in fact. Many exercises consist in attending to the *means* of achieving a goal and not to the goal itself, which is an important way of reducing tension.

All these exercises aim at achieving mental and physical coordination and in particular good erect posture and correct action.

Erect Posture and Correct Action

There is nothing simpler than erect posture; it means a vertical straight line. But all such words, "posture" included, imply something rigid and static. And in fact, indeed, few people do justice to the flexibility of their bodies. On close examination it becomes clear that erect posture is actually dynamic, with the body frame constantly readjusting itself, rather than being held in a fixed and rigid way.

The real advantage of erect posture is ease of rotation around the vertical—that is, from right to left, or the other way around. This rotation widens the human horizon and also is naturally the most frequent movement of the head. During the evolution of the human frame, the most recurrent use made of the head was its turning towards the source of an

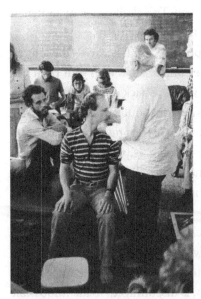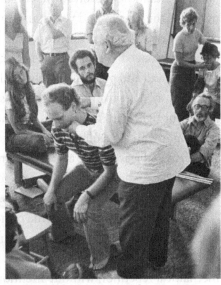

Feldenkrais working with David Zemach-Bersin in the San Francisco training program, 1975.

external stimulus. The senses located in the head all have double organs—vision, hearing, and smell. This is because two sources of data are needed to pinpoint the exact location of the stimulus. For example, the head turns toward a source of sound so that the two ears are equally stimulated. The head also turns to face a visual stimulus. The retinas are internally so connected that they are equally stimulated when we face the object, which originally stimulated one retina more than the other. The same sort of thing happens with odors, though this is a much cruder definition of direction and distance.

Thus our relation with anything outside, beyond what can be explored by the sense of touch, is determined through the movement of the head. All the information from the space around us comes through the head. And our relations with the world outside us affect the quality of the movement of the head most of all.

Numerous mechanisms in the nervous system organize these elementary functions of linkage with the environment, so that when one of the double organs is stimulated, the head rotates until we face the source of the stimulation. The head is rotated on the cervical spine and the twist elongates the skin, muscles, and tendons on the left side of the neck when we turn to the right, and vice versa. The lengthening or stretching of a fiber compresses a nervous fiber inside and this stimulation is used to organize the body so that it is ready to follow the head and face in the direction of the original disturbance in the environment. When the body follows the head, the twist of the neck is undone. The nerve fibers in the muscles of the neck are no longer compressed, and so the body has no more urge to turn.

Like the cervical or neck area, the lower part of the spine is capable of rotating around the central axis. Rotation in the rest of the spine is comparatively small. In both the upper and lower regions of the spine, nerve fibers report rotation of the head to the higher centers, which see to it that the body is so organized that it can rotate to reduce the twist and face in the same direction as the head.

In most people, their heads show clearly with which parts of the space around them they rarely make contact. And the carriage of the head is characteristic of the general bearing and manner of acting of each person.

Another aspect of erect posture is that it is a biological quality of the human frame and there should be no sensation of any doing, holding, or effort whatsoever. For example, the lower jaw with all the teeth has an appreciable weight, yet we have some difficulty in becoming aware that we are doing anything at all to hold up the lower jaw. The *normal* state of the muscles of the lower jaw is a contraction just equal to the gravitational pull on the jaw. Voluntary movements add to or subtract from this permanent contraction. The muscles of the lower jaw, like most skeletal muscles, receive orders in the form of impulses from more than one source. The holding up is assured by antigravity mechanisms in the nervous system and there is no feeling of action, let alone effort, so long as the message to the muscles comes from the lower centers.

In the neck muscles, the same sort of thing obtains. Even though the head is quite heavy and its center of gravity is in front of the spinal column, there is no sensation of effort or action in holding up the head. This is because of the very considerable contraction of certain muscles to hold the head up. The whole body is prevented from falling forward by the calf muscles, but we sense no effort there either. Once again, these relationships show how erect posture is not a static state but a dynamic activity.

Actual posture is always the result of what the frame would do because of inherent mechanisms and of what we have *learned* to do by adjusting ourselves to our physical and social environment. The problem is that much of what we have learned is harmful to our system, because it was learned in childhood, when immediate dependence on others distorted our real needs. Long-standing habitual action *feels* right, but our feeling is unreliable until we re-educate our kinesthetic sense to reality-tested norms. How can this re-education be done? We must first realize the benefits of improvements so that we will spare the needed time. But the benefit cannot be imagined until the improvement is sensed, so at first we must try simply out of curiosity. People whose vitality is at the lowest ebb will not try, and God himself cannot help them.

The body should be so organized that it can start any movement—forward, backward, right, left, down, up, or turning right and left—without previous arrangement of the segments of the body, without any sudden change in the rhythm of breathing, without clenching the lower jaw or tensing the tongue, and without any perceptible tensing of the neck muscles or fixation of the eyes. When the body is organized in this way, the head is not held fixedly but is free to move gently in all directions without previous notice. If these conditions are maintained during an action, then even lifting the entire body is not sensed as an effort. To demonstrate this, bend your right index finger gently and observe the sensation of no effort. Then bend the wrist gently. The effort is the same as that of bending the finger. Now bend the elbow or gently lift the arm, or lower and lift the head or the trunk. In each case the sensation of effort is the same as that of lifting the index finger. But the work done to lift the finger is roughly 100 g cm, that of the wrist, 1,000 g cm, that of the trunk, 500,000 g cm.* When movements are made the sensation of effort does not increase proportionately to the work done, even within such wild limits as 1 to 5,000 and for that matter 1 to a million. This is because the *sensation* of effort does not measure the work done, but indicates the degree of *organization* producing the effort. This organization corresponds to the structure of the body. The size and strength of the muscles increase from the periphery, such as the fingers, to the center of the body. The *rate* of effort is, therefore, equal in all the parts at work. To lift or lower the trunk involves the muscles of the pelvis (such as the buttocks and thigh muscles with their enormous cross-section), as compared with those used in moving the fingers.

Finally, self-knowledge through awareness is the goal of re-education. As we become aware of what we are doing in fact, and not what we *say* or *think* we are doing, the way to improvement is wide open to us.

There is still a vast field left unexplored in the realm of body and mind. But a useful start has been made that provides means to make considerable changes in behavior. There can be no *improvement* without *change*. Though

---

g cm is a notation for grams x centimeters. Here it is indicating the work done (or the amount of torque) and can be thought of as the weight x the lever arm.

For instance, for a finger you have a small weight (roughly 33 g) and a short lever arm (3 cm), since the length of the lever arm is measured from the joint to the finger center-of-mass (i.e., the midpoint of the finger, or half its length). Thus the work in this case is roughly 100 g cm.

help can be given when things go wrong, we cannot relax our effort before teachers throughout the world will learn how to develop in their students awareness of the unity of body and mind so that higher achievements than merely correcting faults can be arrived at. Training a body to perfect all the possible forms and configurations of its members changes not only the strength and flexibility of the skeleton and muscles, but also makes a profound and beneficial change in the self-image and the quality of direction of the self.

3

On the Primacy of Hearing

Three of the most important articles in this collection were first published in English in *Somatics* magazine, edited by Thomas Hanna, PhD (1928–1990). Thomas Hanna was an early supporter and student of Dr. Feldenkrais. He is also credited with helping to coin the term "Somatics" in the 1970s to refer to the emerging field of mind-body approaches. *Somatics: Magazine-Journal of the Bodily Arts and Sciences,* a central venue for the Somatics field, was founded in 1976 by Dr. Hanna, who continued as its editor until his death in 1990. This article was first published in *Somatics* in 1976.*—Ed.*

IN THE DARKNESS OF HUMAN FETAL EXISTENCE, THERE IS LITTLE likelihood that seeing takes place. But even though there is no seeing, there is hearing. The fetus hears the heartbeats of the mother, the noises of her digestive tract, the noises of her breathing, the bubbling of gases, emphysematic disturbances in the breathing tract, or coughing, sneezing, and other noises connected with the digestive tract. There is little doubt that the fetus is stimulated by these many sounds, but we cannot assert that he "hears" them in the way we do: simple response to organic stimulation is very different from the hearing that takes place after personal experience and growth.

This innervation of the ear is a stimulation coming to the fetus from the "outside," just as it later is the case when the baby "sees" the world. But we know that the neonate does not actually see the outside world when he comes into it. Unlike the ears, the eyes have not had any prior stimulation and learning. Indeed, it is generally understood that there is no seeing at all for the first few weeks, even though there is some response to light. It, then, stands to reason that the function of hearing is prior to seeing in each and every individual, just as it is prior in the development of evolutionary structures.

The function of hearing evolved as a response to mechanical vibrations. The ability to respond to finer vibrations, such as oscillations in the air, became true hearing when all of the structural complexity and finesse of the ear and of the nervous system had evolved—function and structure grow and assist each other in this way all along the path of evolutionary development.

An infant is, then, predominantly a hearing animal; the first experience of the world around us is initially sensory and then auditory, even though this slight priority is likely not significant. The first years of a baby's life are passed, not so much in seeing, but in learning to walk and to speak—i.e., the infant is largely sensory and auditory in orientation. A child's memory, its ability to imitate everything it hears, its ability to learn a first language depend on this orientation; later, however, the possibility of learning a second language reflects a greater role played by seeing.

Many people grow up without directly relating their seeing to the outside world; their internal security is based more on their hearing. Such people are especially sensitive to the inflections of the voice. The emotional content of the heard word means more to them than its meaning. In a similar way, most of us prefer to hear a teacher say something rather than read it. Even though the latter way is more exact, hearing makes seeing more concrete and easier to remember and, therefore, to understand. This is the case with our short-term memory, without which we would not be able to relate the end of a sentence to its beginning.

As a child first begins to be trained in reading and writing, his hearing is gradually withdrawn from most of the space around him. He learns to pay increasing attention, sometimes exclusively, to that sector of space which he sees. In general, it is the case that we see only a small part of the space around us, even though in hearing we hear from all around us.

We see here a particular instance of something very general and fundamental: in learning to direct his attention to what his eyes see, the child withdraws his general watchfulness and becomes oblivious to the greater part of the space around him.

Later he will learn to listen to the information of both his ears and eyes. He may already be capable of handling considerable stimulation in both ears and eyes. But he will have to undergo considerably more learning before he will have an undivided attention which can detect minimal or barely perceptible changes. But here again, he will listen—mostly to his ears, checking the eyes for accuracy and detail.

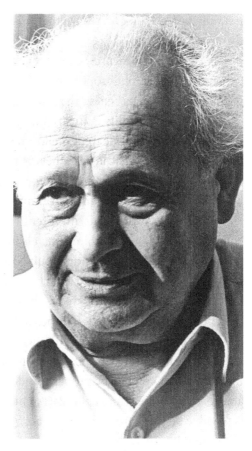

When we arrive in the outside world we have no inkling of what it is. This is because, at first, the stimulation of the senses carries no information other than the fact that the senses are being stimulated. The beginning of our acquaintance with the outside world is not only sensory but is entirely subjective. For a long time we know only a sensorial subjective reality. We are not, however, alone: always we are in communication with other human beings—parents, teachers, etc. Without ever stopping to think about it, we behave as if all these others share the same subjective reality as we.

There are as many subjective realities as there are subjects. The one thing that is common to all these subjective realities is the one reality we use in communicating with one another: the one "objective" reality for all of us.

But, apart from this, there is obviously a third reality. This is Reality—with a capital R—that is understood to exist whether you and I are alive or whether we know it or ignore it. This is the Reality which must exist and must be there, whether men exist or not. When we use our thinking, and not only our sensing, we realize that this third Reality is more than likely the first.

This Reality is immensely complex and is only very superficially known, either to science or philosophy or in music or poetry. But our sense of self-importance makes us believe that our subjective reality is just as valid.

The "objective" reality is, finally, that part of our subjective reality which we are willing to concede to our fellow men. I can see that you can see and that you can read, but I can never believe that you can see as I can, or understand what you read as I do, even though logic forces me to recognize I must be wrong and have no grounds for thinking in this way.

My subjective reality is mine entirely and follows all my whims. "Objective" reality is less whimsical: it is the reality experienced by all men. It limits and restricts your and my subjective reality to that upon which all others agree. Subjective reality is anchored in us and is as real as our bodies. Objective reality is the measure of our sanity. But Reality has never as yet been perceived in its entirety. Our belief that we know Reality is an illusion, a *maya;* it is a measure of our ignorance.

Mind you, I know that our consciousness and awareness can grow. As these functions come to be properly understood and developed, we will be able to bite off, chew, and assimilate a much greater chunk of Reality. This is possible because, from the very start of our lives, our nervous system is not bound by any reality: it is a *tabula rasa* when we come into the world. On a clean board you can write anything, and to make any new writing on the nervous system meaningful and superior, this new writing must be based on our choice and not upon chance.

Each of us comes into the world with a nervous system complete for all the functions necessary to keep that nervous system growing and learning more and more complex activity: all the digestive functions, breathing, eliminatory mechanisms, restoring equilibrium, regulating temperature, heartbeat, maintaining invariant pressures of liquids such as blood, lymph, cerebrospinal fluid, chemical composition, healing and restoring every excessive change back to an optimal homeostatic condition were there—in short, everything that any animal born has in its nervous system—all organized to function and to rebound from accidental changes in functioning.

Many of my clients bring with them a nervous system with parts of it not organized at all. Only the structure is there with no connections to make it function. We have termed this initial state of neural structure—capable of functioning only after personal experience of reality—a *tabula rasa*. Reality helps the structure to organize itself to fit the surrounding medium in which it will have to live. Initially we could not speak any language, we could not walk, we could not read, we could not write, we could not sing, we could not whistle, nor could we yodel. We could not see a three-dimensional object on two-dimensional paper, and we could not count. We had only this *tabula rasa*, capable of being organized to an astonishing facility to accomplish immensely more.

We could, in the beginning, have used our nervous system, the mouth, its muscles, the vocal cords, the feedback from the mouth cavity to the ears and auditory cortex to fit any of the two thousand languages and at least as many dialects with equal facility.

The human species did not start out by being anything but an animal, but ended up becoming the animal *Homo sapiens*. All the other animals come into the world with their structures much more organized to function in almost rigid patterns. Their nervous systems are more complete, and the patterns of connections directing activity are almost set and unalterable but are fit for early action. The *Homo sapiens* animal has a tremendous part of his nervous system left unpatterned, not connected, so that each individual, depending on the environment in which he happens to be born, can organize his brain to fit the surrounding demands. This his brain learns to do. The animal part ready at birth can do only what other animals do. His brain can learn what others can do in only one way, but it can also learn more ways of doing it.

The freedom to learn is a great liability; initially, it also is a restriction. There is no freedom of choice or free will when there is only one way of acting. Learning makes it possible to have alternative ways of performing anything. The ability to learn is synonymous with free choice and free will. But once learned the choice is made, the die is cast, and the *tabula rasa* is no more. Herein lie the liabilities as well as the restriction.

Even as the awareness of being a *Homo sapiens* evolved only gradually, so also the traditional human ways of learning grew gradually and, so to speak, naturally. Traditionally, the process of education was never thought out and the methods which came naturally when dealing with an infant have substantially remained the same. Considering that at the age of two our nervous system attains four-fifths of its ultimate size and weight, everything is basically set and learning will continue on these pre-set lines, in most cases restricting the freedom of learning and choice.

* * *

Most persons with neural malfunctions are not aware that the functions they have lost were originally learned and were not inherited as were their digestion or temperature regulation. Were these latter lost, then life would come to an abrupt end. But these unfortunates have lost learned organization and, like everyone else, they see no difference between the *Homo sapiens* part of themselves and the animal part. They cannot help themselves and neither can anyone else who is not aware of this difference. Many of the evils from which we suffer are rooted in our false understanding that human education is the training of a completed being to do this or that, as if we were making a computer perform a desired activity.

In spite of the apparent darkness of the human future, I believe we have not yet reached our *Homo sapiens* capacities for learning; it is still too early to condemn man on the strength of the small awareness he has acquired by chance and not by his outstanding ability to reduce great complexity to familiar simplicity—in other words, to learn. We have never yet really used our essential freedom of choice and we have barely learned to learn.

It is difficult to choose a suitable example to illustrate the above, but here is a simple one that will show how very much a liability and restriction is our achieved level of learning and how we do not benefit from what our awareness allows us: while in your home or some familiar surrounding, blindfold yourself and live by your ears only. To begin with, do it for only half an hour. You will quickly realize how your awareness is mostly limited to what you can see. Any creature who had to guarantee his individual safety and security could not survive if two-thirds of the space around him was ignored and did not reach awareness.

When we pay attention to what we see we cannot help withdrawing our attention from the better part of the space around us. A wild animal that does not have a samurai-like awareness of what is happening around it and above it cannot endure for long. You and I can do what a trained samurai can do: we can retrain and extend our awareness to the Reality all around us. The ears did just this before their information began to be partially ignored and neglected, and before vision became domineering instead of dominant.

If you continue this demonstration and rely exclusively on your ears for up to a few hours, you will realize how poorly we use ourselves even when our eyes are open. You will notice not only a change toward wider attention but the tonus of your entire being is heightened to buoyancy and freshness. Some esoteric disciplines believe that in such a change the entire consciousness is raised to a higher level. At this level your memory will resemble more what it was during your early childhood before you learned to read. Moreover, your ability to learn and retain will equally improve.

4

On Health

This provocative piece was published in *Dromenon* magazine in 1979. *Dromenon* was a publication connected with Dr. Jean Houston and Dr. Robert Masters, cofounders of the Foundation for Mind Research. Houston and Masters were leaders in the area of consciousness research and the human potential movement. They were friends and early supporters of Dr. Feldenkrais. Houston and Masters authored many books together, including *Mind Games, The Varieties of Psychedelic Experience,* and, in 1978, *Listening to the Body: The Psychophysical Way to Health and Awareness,* based on Feldenkrais's work, for which Dr. Feldenkrais wrote the introduction.—*Ed.*

A healthy person is one who can live fully his unavowed dreams.

A FEW YEARS BEFORE WORLD WAR II, I WAS TEACHING JUDO to make a living while working at the Sorbonne with Joliot-Curie[1] for my doctor's degree in Science. One of my pupils turned out to be a hunter of wild animals in Africa, and he invited me to his house where I was left alone for a few minutes. I was startled when a lion walked in and came over to lick me. It had been brought to Paris as a cub and had grown up into a real lion.

A few months later the lion was taken by the police to the Paris Zoo. The lion had gone into the street and an old lady with a little Pekingese dog and dim eyesight, mistaking him for a big dog, chased him through the streets with her umbrella. After refusing food and drink for about ten days, the lion died in its cage. I have shortened the story by omitting the details.

Now, there was a healthy animal that died, obviously due to an emotional trauma. But what is a healthy animal? If a healthy lion dies ten days after a sudden change in its life, what is health?

If a human being needs no medical services for years and has no complaints of pains or aches, is he or she healthy? If, on the other hand, this same person leads a dull, uninteresting life with marital difficulties that end up with suicide—is that a healthy person? And is a person who never brings his or her work to an end one way or another, and who keeps changing his employment only to avoid his duties time and time again—is he in good health?

Obviously, health is not easy to define. It is certainly not enough to say that not asking for medical or psychiatric help is proof of health.

What, then, is health?

Life is a process. This means that whatever goes on in us while we are alive is linked with time. Everybody knows that, even if nobody thinks or says so. A process cannot be stopped for any length of time, depending on the forces that are involved. And of course everybody knows that if the brain does not get oxygen for ten or fifteen seconds, the process stops altogether. If one succeeds in restarting it by chance, it is a new process and the person is never again what he was. If a person bleeds enough he bleeds to death, and a heart that stopped for that reason is not easy to set working again. In short, any process stopped, will not start again spontaneously. This is true of any irreversible chemical process or of any reaction.

So, obviously, health means first of all that all the essential functions of a person must be able to continue without prolonged breaks. Consciousness, the central nervous system, the heart, and so on have to go on uniformly. There is nothing here that we don't really know.

Very large systems that function are also processes depending on time. Any of the very large companies or any nation are good examples: Ford, ICI, Philips, or any such large system. All such systems will continue functioning no matter which particular factory, mine, or city ceases to exist. The measure of a large system is the size of the shock it can take without its processes stopping.

Now, the human nervous system has 3.10 (10)* parts at least. This is a system large enough for its balanced functions to obey the law of large systems. The health of such a system can be measured by the shock it can take without compromising the continuation of its process. In short, health is measured by the shock a person can take without his usual way of life being compromised.

The usual way of life thus becomes the criterion of health. Sleep, food, breathing, changes of weather, cold, heat, work should all be capable of large variations—sudden shocks. The healthier the person, the more easily will he regain the conduct of his life after considerable sudden shocks by changes in all the necessities for life.

On reflection there is nothing here that is very difficult to accept, except that we may be surprised to find where this leads us. Our nervous system is not born as it is when we are adults. In order to get a system to work as it does in us, the nervous system needs the outside world. There is light of different intensities and colors. Objects are near or farther away, and so on. Our eyes therefore first have to learn to see, even a three-dimensional object in a two-dimensional picture. In short, our system needs a special part of the world to learn a language.

But there are more fundamental issues. The system is wired-in through its sensory and kinesthetic organs to the external world. A non-differentiated nervous system, while it grows, gets differentiated to cope finely with outside objects. What does this entail in a practical sense?

It means that we have to learn to separate functionally—i.e., to differentiate our senses from feelings. A baby seeing a red object has a feeling of red, since the object has no meaning unless you are grown up and know what the object is. Hearing a drum for the first time produces a feeling of something startling, a feeling of a kinesthetic jolt. Only later, having had many jolts of the kind, a differentiation of the sensation and the audible

---

*It is not clear from the original text what number was meant to be used here. Many very large numbers are used to try to express the complexity of the nervous system. One estimate used today is 100 billion neurons in a human brain and 100 trillion synapses.

sense will result in hearing and perceiving a drum. The same sort of differentiation of the kinesthetic feeling from external objects, which may affect our taste, tactile experiences, our smell, and the senses we have already discussed, will gradually occur.

All such differentiations do not happen to all the senses uniformly, and each baby has of course an entirely individual history of development, so that some people conceive the outside world preferably visually, some audibly, some tactually or kinesthetically. In reality most people have their senses and feelings differentiated to different degrees.

It is perhaps not self-evident that all of us can visualize or hear an object when we imagine it or when we recall the experiences which produced the differentiation. This applies equally to the other senses.

In the end it is this learning to know the outside world through our senses which forms our nervous system. A long, complicated learning process like this cannot be perfect nor error-free in all people. Just as there are all sorts of fish in the sea, there are all sorts of people in the world. Some will grow and form their own way of relating to the world in conditions of security, with a good heredity and at different periods of the growth of human civilization and culture. Others are not so lucky.

Some of the tendencies of every one of us will remain tendencies for as long as we live. They have never been differentiated to be of any practical use in acting and reacting in the world around us … everyone has his unavowed dreams when grown up. Our culture, parents, and schooling make us dismiss these dreams as infantile attitudes not befitting a realistic adult. We gradually suppress them, are somehow ashamed to be very serious about them. But luckily not all of us. Some exceptionally fortunate ones succeed even to the point of making them come true—and some find their inspiration in other occupations just by avoiding taking their dreams seriously.

I am not sure that I have made the problem clear enough. Let me say, however, that the healthy person is the one who can live his unavowed dreams fully. There are healthy people among us, but not very many.

In our culture, the life process, starting with a widening of the differentiation of the nervous system to a finer and more complete variety of expe-

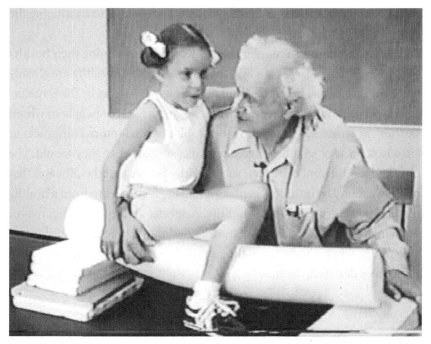

Feldenkrais helping a child learn to walk.

riences of the outside world, with an increased ability to change it for our growing intentional activity, slows and narrows its scope with sexual maturity. After that the system narrows its links with the external world as a whole and specializes in a particular aspect of the external phenomena. We become expert in a narrowing peak of activities and experience. We become a poet, a boxer, a scientist, a politician, a painter, a musician, an economist, a surgeon, a dancer—the choice is interminable. Our learning is then not concerned directly with continuing the essential differentiation of the nervous system through a widening commerce with the outside world.

There comes a point where our education as it developed does not help us, but very often limits and directs us into channels which are not conducive to health. We become so unhealthy that we have to retire before we are biologically old—we are simply unhealthy. Some bits of us—those involved in the peak formation of our activity—are worn out. The life process is narrowed. Activity is restricted more and more to the specialty in which we excel. Only those parts of the nervous system essential to continuing the process of biological existence function, after a fashion.

Even in our culture a number of us succeed in continuing their healthy life process to an old age—an age, that is, where the unhealthy are already dotty and sick. Some of our best and healthiest men—who, by the way, may be hunchbacks or have other deformities—are the sort of people of whom we think as artists. Most artists, be they cobblers or sculptors, composers or virtuosos, poets or scientists, like good wine, are best when they are old. The outstanding difference between such healthy people and the others is that they have found by intuition, genius, or had the luck to learn from a healthy teacher, that learning is the gift of life. A special kind of learning: that of knowing oneself. They learn to know "how" they are acting and thus are able to do "what" they want—the intense living of their unavowed, and sometimes declared, dreams.

5

Man and the World

This article is based on a talk given at the Explorers of Humankind conference in Los Angeles in 1978. Other speakers included Alexander Lowen, Ida Rolf, Charlotte Selver, Charles Brooks, Carl Rogers, Karl Pribram, and Margaret Mead. In 1979 a book based on the conference, *Explorers of Humankind,* was edited by Thomas Hanna, and this piece was included there. It was also published in *Somatics* magazine the same year. *–Ed.*

CONSISTING OF AN ASTRONOMICAL NUMBER OF CELLS, the human nervous system is fit to live and function in a great variety of physical worlds. As the experience of so many astronauts has shown, our nervous system can stand up to a lack of gravitation and to the practical absence of both auditory and visual stimulation. In order to maintain awareness at its normal level, it was enough for the astronauts to initiate activities in which a sufficient number of successive cues occurred at close intervals.

I believe that our nervous system would function well in a thousand different possible worlds. It would grow and adapt itself, or better still, it would learn to act and respond to any conditions in which life can exist. Because it seeks order and consistency, our nervous system can, for example, be "wired-in" to cope easily with any of the three thousand languages and as many dialects that exist on earth.

The cosmos (meaning "order," in Greek) is not very predictable except for a few things like day and night, lunar phases, and the seasons. I am not sure that simpler nervous systems are aware even of these orderly phenomena. Otherwise, randomness is the rule. Meteorites have a very disorderly way of falling. No one can predict which atom will disintegrate at a given moment in any radioactive material. The falling of a particular raindrop at a precise place and instant is anybody's guess. The situation is the same with earthquakes, winds, typhoons, suns, and galaxies, as well as on the microscopic level with solids, gases, or liquids. Whatever we may choose for examination, there is little that is predictable, orderly, stable, and invariant. In most phenomena too many parameters are involved to detect cause and effect, which means to us, order.

But nervous structures look for order and will find it when and where it can be found or can be asserted. Only nervous systems, consisting of such great numbers of units as there are in most living creatures, need consistency and constancy of environment. To form a self, to find a mate, to live in a herd, flock, or society it is imperative to have an organization that is repetitive so that it will be possible to learn to cope with the world. For the more complex life forms—monkeys swinging from one branch to another thirty feet away or humans playing tennis or violins—it is essential for them to form sets of invariants which allow learning while growing. This is a type of learning quite apart from academic learning.

All living creatures, when born, are smaller and weaker than their grown-up parents, some for shorter and some for longer intervals of time. Weak organisms need a consistent and constant world in order to grow into strong adults. As we know, an organism is within itself an entire world of micro-beings which needs, in its turn, a consistent outside world so that the internal world can have homeostasis, order, and invariance, a condition that must be maintained if it is to exist at all for any length of time.

In short, a living nervous system introduces order into the random, constantly changing stimuli arriving through the senses and impinging on the system. Moreover, the living organism itself is moving incessantly, and the nervous system has to bring order to the mobile, changing world, as well as to its own mobility, to make some sense from this whirling turmoil.

Quite surprisingly, the most efficient means for achieving this Herculean feat is *movement*. Movement of the living organism is essential for the formation of *stationary* events in the changing, moving environment and the constantly moving organism itself. Even if we are observing inert matter, our senses still perceive moving impressions, since a living organism is never completely stationary until it dies.

Professor Heinz von Foerster[1] of the Biological Computer Laboratory, a cyberneticist who nourishes similar ideas, has noted that the French mathematician Henri Poincaré[2] wrote in 1887 that three-dimensional vision is possible not only because there are two eyes but also because of the movement of the head which carries them. The head movements need the adjustment of the eyes, and three-dimensional pictures would not be perceived with eyes that were merely stationary in space.

Van Foerster has also told of a Swiss ski instructor, Köhler,[3] who persuaded some of his pupils to participate in a fascinating experiment. He wanted to find out what would happen if our brain saw the outside world as it is on the retina and not as it actually is. As everyone knows, the eye lens, like any other lens, inverts the image on the retina. When seen, a standing person has his head at the bottom of the retina and his feet at the top. Mr. Köhler gave all the participants a pair of glasses inverting the image on the retina to be the right way up. As expected, he and all the others saw everything upside down. The first hours were very difficult; nobody could move freely or do anything without going very slowly and trying to figure out and make sense of what they saw. Then something unexpected happened:

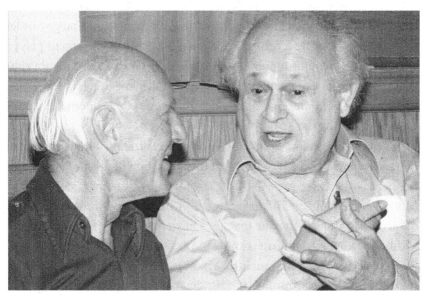

Feldenkrais with Heinz von Foerster 1977.

Everything about their bodies and the immediate vicinity that they were touching began to look as before, but everything which could not be touched continued to be inverted. Gradually, by groping and touching while moving around to attain the satisfaction of normal needs, objects farther afield began to appear normal to the participants in the experiment. In a few weeks, everything looked the right way up, and they could all do everything with-out any special attention or care. At one point in the experiment snow began to fall. Mr. Köhler looked through the window and saw the flakes rising from the earth and moving upwards. He went out, stretched his hands, palms upwards, and felt the snow falling on them. After only a few moments of feeling the snow touch his palms, he began to see the snow falling instead of rising.

There have been other experiments with inverted spectacles. One car-ried out in the USA involved two people, one sitting in a wheelchair and the other pushing it, both being fitted with such special glasses. The one who moved around by pushing the chair began to see normally and, after a few hours, was able to find his way without groping, while the one sitting con-tinued to see everything the wrong way.

Does a newborn baby see the right way from the start? Or does he, instead, have to move and touch things in order to be able to interpret and give order to the impressions he receives? I, for one, suspect that movement plays a central role in forming our objective world. And, if my suspicion is not alto-gether wrong, movement may be necessary for all living things to form their orderly, objective, exterior world and perhaps even their internal image of the world.

One thing is certain: We are not merely the realization of the program of our given genetic code. We know that the realization of this program never happens without the growth of the organism bearing that genetic code. Moreover, being born and growing never happens without at least one observer or witness—the one that gives birth to the new organism. And, in addition, no living organism is known to exist outside a gravitational field.

In sum, a genetic program is incorporated into a body that grows from two cells to whatever number of cells, in an environment inevitably situ-ated in a gravitational field that is never without witnesses. None of these items—the genetic code, the witnesses, and the gravitational field—can alone, by any stretch of the imagination, form a living being able to grow and become adult.

All mammals have skeletons, muscles, and nervous systems, and they are born to parents, and the earth exercises on all of them the same gravitational force that is never interrupted and cannot be screened. Man, being a mammal, shares this same estate. There are, however, important differences. The human skeleton has the thumbs so structured that he can touch the tips of all of his fingers. An orangutan or chimpanzee has power-producing muscles in its arms stronger than man, but the fine musculature of the human hand allows for a manipulative range of extreme finesse. Think of writing, making music, watchmaking, etc. The functional differences of the nervous system of man mark him apart from all other mammals. Parenthood in man is also very different. A human child usually has a father and a mother, plus two grandfathers and two grandmothers. The human environment involves the self and the self-image as well as the sexual, the social, and cultural, besides the spatial and temporal aspects of it.

The movements involved in every action produce a displacement of the entire organism with changes in its configuration, all of which affect different aspects of the environment in order to provide for the necessities of the organism. There is, then, a continuously changing environment with a continuously changing organism, both interacting without cease, so long as there is life in the organism. Different environments affect the organism and the nervous system so as to cause it to act and react effectively and efficiently to these changes.

We have then, from birth till death, a closed loop of four elements: skeleton, muscles, nervous system, and environment. These elements are, in fact, very complex systems interacting with numerous feedbacks and feedforwards all along the loop. The loop can be drawn as a quadrangle with four sides and four summits. In my own work I deal mostly with the summits rather than with the sides. I deal with the linkage at the summits where the elements interact with one another and where the learned use of self is more apparent. The individual life of intentional activity and reacting can more easily be changed through learning than through the more rigid structures represented by the sides—i.e., bones, muscles, nervous system, space-culture-time, etc. It is also better to improve the way we do things than what we do. For *how* we do something is often more important than *what* we do.

These four complex elements can be studied from the beginning of life to the end. At birth the organism/environmental link is largely passive. By and by, passivity is replaced by more and more intentional activity. Were there no gravitation the whole scheme would be radically different. Bones would not be built to withstand compression. Velocity and power of movements would be different. It would be something that we could hardly conceive. As it is, movement is the best clue to life. Ever since man could speak he classified all existing things according to their movement in the gravitational field. Vegetation is everything which moves passively from side to side, following the flow of water or air; otherwise, its growth is vertical. Living things are classified after the way they move. The swimming ones are fishes, the flying ones are birds, the gliding ones are snakes, the wriggling ones are worms. There are jumping ones, crawling ones, the ones who walk on all fours, and we, featherless bipeds, who walk upright. Movement seems to have preoccupied man since he could first remember himself.

Movement is central to each living cell making up the organism, and the whole of it—the skeleton, the muscles, and the nervous system—is preoccupied with movement. The organization of movement is so complex that most living things need some personal individual apprenticeship, be they fishes, birds, apes, or men. The amount of apprenticeship varies from a few seconds or minutes to many years. Some of the herd animals, especially the bovines, horses, zebras, and their like, seem to be able to follow the herd almost immediately after they are dropped by the mother cow, mare, or whatever. The newborn will make an attempt or two to get on its feet immediately after its umbilical cord is chewed and it is licked all over. When the second or third attempt at standing is successful, the calf will follow the cow on sand, gravel, or slippery wet grass, no matter whether it is on level, ascending, or descending ground. It can not only do everything necessary to cling to the herd, but if it happens to slide or stumble it can right itself. If one thinks of the complexity and ingenuity necessary to construct a machine that is similarly efficient, one can realize what is involved in this extraordi-

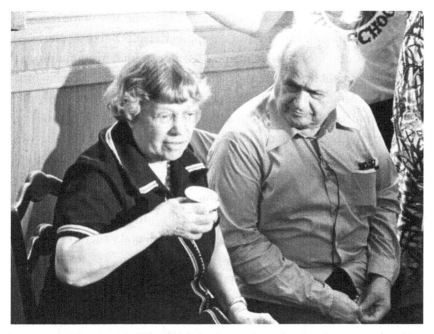

Feldenkrais with anthropologist Margaret Mead, 1977.

nary ability to move without previous experience and with so little apprenticeship.

Think of the mountain goats, where the kids are born on high rocks. The kids right themselves on their feet and then have to leap from one sharp edge to another without previous apprenticeship. Obviously, all the connections, the "wiring-in," of the nervous systems of these animals must be made before they are born. In short, with nonhuman animals, it is the species that has handed down the learning, the evolving, the reflex organization, the instinct which enables them to survive in precarious conditions. However, most birds, dogs, kittens of all sorts, even tiger kittens, have to have some kind of coaching by their parents to finish the "wiring-in," establishing the functioning patterns of their nervous systems. That which can make this pattern reliable, autonomous, or automatic needs an apprenticeship of a few weeks.

When we pass in review many of the species, it becomes evident that: the *lower* a species' place on the ladder of evolution, the more complete is the wiring-in of the nervous system at birth. The connection of the synapses, neurons, or whatever is ready and the apprenticeship is shorter, the lower the species are on the ladder. In man, we see the extreme end of this process. The human infant has, to my knowledge, the longest apprenticeship of all the species. Although everything necessary to maintain life and growth is already connected in the nervous and glandular systems at birth, the specific human functions are not wired-in at all. No baby was ever born who could speak, sing, whistle, crawl, walk upright, make music, count or think mathematically, or tell the hour of the day or night. Without a very long apprenticeship lasting several years, none of these functions has ever been observed to develop. As far as these specifically human functions or activities go, the connections or the wiring-in of the neural structures are non-existent at birth.

It is the individual, personal experience or apprenticeship that is necessary and without it the baby will not be a human being. It is as if there were no inherited learning in the human species whatsoever. The "lower" animals have phylogenetic learning—the inherited and evolved learning of their species. The "higher" animal learns through his own individual onto-genetic experience. The "lower" and "higher" have little meaning other than to refer to the complexity of our way of putting together the ladder of evolution. Almost all the lower animals can do things that the highest can never do without prolonged learning, and then only through imitation, usually with a great variety of auxiliary instruments or structures.

The tendency to repetition leads in the end to repetitive constancy and order. Most happenings are ruled by chance and are so disorderly that most goings-on are not predictable. We make the laws of nature by singling out the parts of events to which we can add what we consider order. Newton made order in an impressive array of disorderly falling bodies by promoting gravitation to the status of being. Only nervous tissues and systems are capable of conceiving and realizing. In human beings it is the neural substance that organizes order in its own functioning; it makes order in its environment, which in turn improves the orderliness of the human, and so on. The neural substance organizes itself and thereby selects and alters the incoming messages from the environment into invariant sets, thus making

66

repetition possible. Many continuously changing messages are received from the environment before the organism succeeds in perceiving them as unchanging entities. So great is the ability of the nervous system that it creates order where instruments made of any other matter will register a blur or continuous variations. Just think of taking a photograph of a greyhound running toward you while you are sitting on a galloping horse. We can understand each other while a fan or an air conditioner makes so much background noise that no recorder will reproduce an intelligible record of what we said. We have no difficulty extracting invariant order out of many varying interferences. In anything we see, hear, smell, or feel, we actively organize ourselves so as to be impressed by those invariant sets that allow us to cope with the disorder both within ourselves and outside ourselves in the environment, whether interpersonal, social, spatial, or temporal.

Put simply: a thing is alive if it has a boundary separating it from the rest of the world, if it can reproduce itself, if it can maintain itself (i.e., draw energy from outside its boundary), and if it can preserve itself. All these functions cannot occur without self-direction—i.e., movement. The widening of awareness through movement is a learning process that has been used ever since the first cell took on a membrane, becoming an individual needing to direct itself.

Awareness Through Movement is a learning process that makes self-direction easier and more pleasurable, because it resembles the learning that occurs with growth itself. The two methods I use, *Awareness Through Movement* and *Functional Integration,* are essentially an efficient, short, and general way of *learning to learn.* In traditional learning it is *what* we learn that is important. But the higher function of learning to learn is free of such restrictions. Learning to learn involves an improvement of the brain function itself which carries it beyond its latent potential.

To facilitate such learning it is necessary to divorce the aim to be achieved from the learning process itself. The process is the important thing and should be aimless to the adult learner just as is learning to the baby. The baby is not held to any timetable nor is there any need to rely on force. Re-education of the adult has been corrupted by the teaching methods traditionally learned in schools and by academic teaching in general. In both, the teacher is presumed to be superior to the learner and is an example to follow and to imitate. Achievement is the aim, not learning; and precise times are fixed for specific achievements. Learning such as this has nothing to do with growth: it can be delayed at will or even abandoned altogether. But the learning that is dependent on growth cannot be delayed with impunity, nor can it be accelerated beyond the normal pace of growth.

I believe that the possibility of a better future for humanity is nearer to our grasp than is presumed by the gloomy outlook of self-destruction that is predicted and held by many. A society in which its members are only so many units composing it, is not the final form of society. A society of men and women with greater awareness of themselves will, I believe, be one that will work for the human dignity of its members rather than primarily for the abstract, collective notion of human society.

6

Awareness Through Movement

This short and concise piece includes both theory and concrete descriptions of Feldenkrais's educational approach. It was used as a handout at his Institute in Tel Aviv. This version, published in the *Annual Handbook for Group Facilitators* in 1975, varies only slightly from the article used at the Institute.—*Ed.*

MAN IS AN ANIMAL BECAUSE OF HIS STRUCTURE. But he is the highest animal and a human being because of the functioning of his nervous system. The hand of man differs only slightly from that of an ape in the position and movement of the thumb—but the nervous system of man allows him to use the muscles and bones of his hand to do what an anthropoid ape cannot do: the fine, manipulative, specifically human movements such as writing, playing an instrument, counting bank notes, repairing a watch, or focusing a microscope.

Two Modes of Learning

Learning the two uses of the hand happens in two different modes. The common movements of the hands are spontaneous and improve with the growth of every normal animal—ape or man. The fine, human, manipulative skills, however, must be taught to every individual human being in a specific way and at a proper time.

The specific mode of learning (perhaps the most important property of the human nervous system) is apparent not only in man's hands but in all his functions. Man's upright stance, his gait, his speech—all are learned and need several years of apprenticeship and then many more years to achieve perfection.

The ability to utter noises (i.e., the animal part of speech) improves with growth in both man and other mammals, but a person who grows to be an adult outside a human society may never reach the skill of an average human being. Animal instinct is *phylogenetic* learning, or the learning of the species; human learning is *ontogenetic*—i.e., it needs personal experience. In short, learning is to the human nervous system what instinct is to animals.

Dogs, for instance, learn spontaneously all canine languages, and a Chinese dog can communicate with an American dog as well as with a Persian one. But a human nervous system "wired-in" through personal, individual experience can speak only one language. The remaining two thousand or so tongues will remain forever foreign unless the individual engages in new learning.

Instinct has certain drawbacks, as does human learning. Instinct is useless in a suddenly changed environment or a completely new situation. The value of learning depends on the choice and the quality of what is learned. The human nervous system, however, in which the patterns of actions are wired-in during the learning process and are not inherited (as are instincts), has a major advantage: relearning or re-education is comparatively easy.

Movement

The best clue to the activity of the human nervous system is movement. Tremors, paralysis, ataxia, impeded speech, and poor muscular control generally indicate injury or derangement of the function of the brain stem or other parts of the nervous system. Movement or its absence shows the state of the nervous system, its hereditary endowment, and its degree of development. Movement occurs only when the nervous system sends the impulses that contract the necessary muscles in the right patterns or assemblies and in the right sequences in time.

When born, we can do very little voluntary movement besides crying and contracting all the flexors in an undifferentiated effort. We learn by experience how to roll, crawl, sit up, walk, speak, run, jump, balance, rotate, and do whatever else we are capable of performing as adults.

Our consciousness becomes gradually adjusted to our surrounding environment. The first contacts with the outside world are through the skin and mouth. Later we learn to use the parts of our bodies separately and regulate them through seeing them. The major difficulty is differentiation of movements. Thus the fourth finger will remain clumsy unless we play an instrument or make a special point of learning to move it at will. Usually, however, we manage to bring the all-or-none response of the primitive muscular contraction to a more or less perfectly differentiated voluntary activity. Normally, we arrive at this naturally—i.e., without being aware of the process involved, or of the state or degree of perfection achieved in our apprenticeship. The majority of us achieve a happy-go-lucky mediocrity, just enough to make us one of the many.

The *Feldenkrais Method*

My technique of bringing about better maturation of our nervous system uses the reversible relationship of our muscular and nervous systems. Both have evolved in the gravitational field, which sets the standard both for the development and apprenticeship of each individual and also for the evolution of the species.

The extraordinary development of the frontal lobes in man shows that the functioning of these is an evolutionary improvement and helps the survival of the fittest. This development of the human brain becomes effective through its growth after birth and is thus directed and molded through personal individual experience.

Opportunity and Vulnerability

As a result, man has both the extraordinary opportunity—given to no other animal—to build up a body of learned responses and the special vulnerability of going wrong. Since other animals have their responses to most stimuli wired-in to their nervous systems in the form of instinctive patterns of action, they go wrong less frequently.

Even more irritating, we have little opportunity to become aware of where we went wrong. Since we are the learner and the judge at the same time, our judgment depends on, and is limited to, our learning achievements.

Obviously, to improve, we individuals have to better our judgment. But judgment is the result of learning already completed.

Increase in Sensitivity

To break this vicious circle, we must use the basic quality of the supralimbic part of our brain, which is able to sense and abstract and often even express in words what is happening in our bodies. By reducing all stimuli to their bare minimum, we also reduce to its lowest value any change in our muscular system and senses. We thus increase our sensitivity to its maximum and can therefore distinguish the finer details that escaped our notice before. We are like a color-blind person to whom the ability to differentiate between red and green has been restored.

Once the ability to differentiate is improved, the details of the self or the surroundings can be better sensed; we become aware of what we are doing and not what we say or think we are doing.

Lessons in the Method

To begin with, the lessons take place in the lying position, prone or supine, to facilitate the breaking down of muscular patterns. The habitual pressures on the soles of the feet and the ensuing configuration of the skeletal joints are suppressed. The nervous system does not receive the habitual afferent stimuli due to gravitation, and the efferent impulses are not linked into the habitual patterns. After the lessons, on receiving again the habitual stimuli, one is surprised to discover a changed response to them.

The lessons are done as slowly and pleasantly as possible, with no strain or pain whatsoever; the main object is not to receive training in what one knows, but to discover unknown reactions in oneself and thereby learn a better, more congenial way of acting.

The movements are light, so that after fifteen or twenty repetitions the initial effort drops to practically nothing more than a thought. This produces the maximum sensitivity in the person and enables him to detect the minute changes in the efferent tonus and the change in alignment of the different parts of the body.

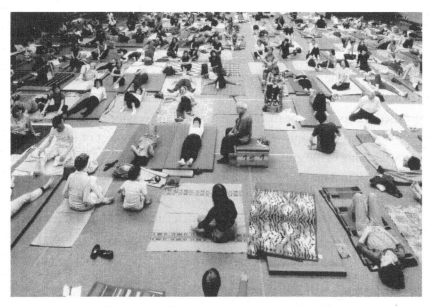

Seminar in 1981, Freiburg in Breisgau, Germany.

By the end of the lessons, one feels that his body is hanging lightly from his head, his feet do not stamp on the ground, and his body glides when moving.

The head, which carries all the teleceptors—eyes, ears, nostrils, and mouth—and which turns right and left in almost every movement, attending to changes in the space around us, should turn with a smoothness unequaled by the most perfect man-made mechanism. Of all the teleceptors, the eyes also move right and left, relative to the head, and their movement in the direction of the head's rotation or opposite to it should be gliding and easy.

Results

Training a body to perfect all the possible forms and configurations of its members not only changes the strength and flexibility of the skeleton and muscles, but makes a profound change in the self-image and the quality of direction of the self.

Two Major Techniques

The Method employs a manipulative and a group technique. The manipulative technique is necessarily individual and is custom tailored to fit the particular needs of the person. About thirty different positions of the body are used. Historically, the manipulative technique was the first to be evolved.

The group technique was created to produce the effect of the manipulative teaching in the greatest possible number of people. (The word *teaching* indicates that the changes in self-image are produced by the pupil through becoming aware of his changed body image.) Lessons have been broadcast by Swiss Radio Zürich for two years. To date, nearly a thousand lessons of forty-five minutes each exist in Hebrew and a few hundred in English, French, and German.

Application of the Method

By seeing all functioning as a manifestation of the nervous system, the *Feldenkrais Method* has universal applicability. I have taught world-famous musicians, violinists, and pianists, such as the well-known conductor Igor Markevitch,[1] who has used my services in the international course of orchestra conductors in Salzburg and in the opera of Monte Carlo for many years. In the last few years I have taught yearly for Peter Brook[2] in his International Centre for Theatre Research in Paris, as well as in San Juan Bautista, where he worked with El Teatro Campesino, and at the Brooklyn Academy of Music. The drama faculties of Carnegie-Mellon University, the University of Pittsburgh, New York University, and many others have used my techniques. I have also done work with chronic ailments and deficiencies.

References

Darwin, C. R. *Expressions of the Emotions in Man and Animals.* New York: AMS Press, 1972.

Feldenkrais, M. *Body and Mature Behavior.* New York: International Universities Press, 1970.

Feldenkrais, M. *Awareness Through Movement: Health Exercises for Personal Growth.* New York: Harper & Row, 1972.

Pribram, K. H. *Languages of the Brain.* (Experimental Psychology Series.) Englewood Cliffs, NJ: Prentice Hall, 1971.

Young, J. Z. *An Introduction to the Study of Man.* New York: Oxford University Press, 1974.

7

Self-Fulfillment Through Organic Learning

Edited by Mark Reese

Dr. Feldenkrais presented this talk at the San Diego Mandala Conference in 1981. The conference that year focused on holistic health and longevity. Mark Reese (1951–2006), part of the original group of students Dr. Feldenkrais trained in the United States, arranged for Dr. Feldenkrais to present at the conference and later edited the talk for publication. Reese went on to become one of the most influential and articulate members of his generation of Feldenkrais teachers and was responsible for training large numbers of new Feldenkrais teachers worldwide. Mark has written a much-anticipated biography of Feldenkrais, *Moshe Feldenkrais: A Life in Movement,* which will be published in 2011.–Ed.

I USUALLY DON'T MAKE IT TO CONFERENCES. I TALK TO PEOPLE and I feel like talking to friends. As a lecturer, I'm not a lecturer. I just talk to people who would like to learn something. I'm not an ordinary teacher either, but a peculiar sort of teacher who is interested not in his teaching but in what people learn. Therefore, I never, never wrote or prepared a lecture in my life. There are many people of the *Feldenkrais* GUILD® here who know me and will witness that for four or eight years of teaching I never prepared anything. This time I wrote a paper, and of course, I don't need it.

I wrote this because I didn't know what I undertook, that the name of my talk should be "Self-Fulfillment Through Organic Learning." About "organic learning" I could talk without preparing, but "self-fulfillment"— what is self-fulfillment? I never can do anything with abstract notions without talking for days and getting nowhere. I need concrete things that are plausible to everyone, that you and I can understand, and that we can touch, see, or hear. After that, when we have some common experience, we can understand one another when we use language. Otherwise, it's impossible. I can say a word like "holistic" and you understand God knows what by that word. What is it? I learned the word "holistic" like Dr. Lomas said yesterday, from Field Marshal Smuts'[1] book. Since then I have seen the word so used and misused that I don't know what it means anymore.

I must begin with concrete things. What is self? What is fulfillment? What is organic learning? If we don't know what we are talking about, we will get nowhere. So first let's see: What is a self? There are four and a half billion selves, and there are not two of them equal, neither in their fingerprints, nor in their immune system. We cannot transplant things from one person to another; they are individuals, each one absolutely unique in his own right. That's a self. This is a simple sort of thing. But there are probably two hundred billion selves like that in the world because all the animals are also selves. What are common to all these selves are very fundamental biological quantities or qualities.

First, self-reproduction. Without self-reproduction no species can exist. All species that exist, including man, must be able to reproduce themselves. The next is self-maintenance. There is no animal, no bacteria, no creature in the world which can exist without absorbing either oxygen, or nitrogen, like the anaerobic bacteria. And water is essential to all life, and food. Without self-maintenance it's inconceivable that any species could exist for a long time. In fact, maintenance is much more drastic than self-reproduction because self-reproduction occurs no more than once or twice a year for most mammals. But maintenance—if you don't breathe for two, three minutes, you won't breathe forever after. Self-preservation is even more drastic: not to be eaten up by a lion or a boa constrictor; falling from a rock, or a high mountain, or a precipice. This can be a question of a second and you're not there. These three "selfs"—self-preservation, self-maintenance, and self-reproduction—are common to all animals; they have nothing to do with human beings alone. None of these three selfs can be satisfied without self-propulsion, or movement, or action. You can't self-reproduce without movement; if you don't move nothing will happen. And you cannot get your food, air, and water without moving. You cannot avoid dangers and preserve yourself without running away, attacking, or being careful in the movement you do—whatever you learned how to do so you could survive.

Although this is common to all living creatures on this earth, the human being is complicated by extraordinary things like thinking, feeling, sensing, consciousness, awareness. What are these things? With what are we going to deal? Awareness, consciousness. Consciousness is also common to most animals, but to such a minor degree, and the difference with which we are endowed with it is so great that you can say it's a different quality. When I ask most people why they have to have consciousness, they say it's enough to be awake. You sleep, you're awake; what do you want to have consciousness for? And in fact, what do you do with your consciousness? What is it? Isn't being awake enough? Well, it turns out that it isn't, because you yourself can see through personal experience; for instance, you can wake up and not know where you are, and not know whether you are awake or not. You can take a child out of his bed and take him to urinate because you want the bed to remain dry. The child gets up and obviously he does feel that he's getting up. He's awake and he's doing something and going back to bed, but he is not conscious; he doesn't know anything and he doesn't even remember that he was lifted out of bed.

So to be awake is not being conscious. What is it, then, to be conscious? When you are unconscious, say, after a car accident, or wake up in a hospital not knowing where you are, the first thing you say is "Where am I?" This is actually one of the essences of consciousness. Before you are oriented in the gravitational field so that you know whether you're sitting or standing, and that your eyes meet the horizon in the normal way, you don't know whether you're asleep, whether you are dreaming, whether you're sitting, whether you are standing, whether you are folding your arms or not. This is one of the major problems of consciousness: to know where you are, what you are doing.

Now what's the difference between consciousness and awareness? Just to repeat: Consciousness has to do with your orientation in the gravitational field. Without that you don't know where you are, what you are, what you are doing, or what is happening with you. Awareness is being conscious and knowing something about it. For instance, I look at you here and I know you are you, but if you ask me how many people are here, I don't know. I have to count them. What do I do to count them? Actually an internal sort of thing. I shift my eyes to you, and I say one and two, then three; I count my own shifts of attention. Then I want to know how many ladies sit here and how many men. Again I shift attention. If I want to count peas, it's the same thing. In other words, counting is an internal affair. Very funny. We think we count oranges; but in fact, whether we count oranges, peas, human beings, or anything, we count the number of shifts of attention of the eyes or the ears. I will show you some very interesting, almost incredible, things, once you know what we are going to come to. Awareness is a question of knowing what you're doing, knowing what you are conscious of. Now we've said something about the "selfs," which, of course, is only roughly touching the thing. If you want to know what the self is really, there are many psychologies and theories. My own approach is quite different from what other people do.

Now, what is fulfillment? Fulfill what? I say that if I want to know what fulfillment is I can get to it only if I know what the *limitations* of fulfillment are. Otherwise, fulfillment of what? Fulfillment of four thousand or four billion people's consciousness, or what? What do they want? Everyone wants something else. Then how? *How* does he or she want something else? By the limitations we can understand the thing. Let's see how the limitations come about.

The human being is born a *tabula rasa*. The minor abilities that he has coming into the world out of his mother's womb are practically insignificant. He can't do any of the things that most animals can do in a few days or weeks. For him, the whole thing is concerned with an experience of learning. What can he do? Most of the things like sweating, say, the animal functions of the body, he has more or less under control within a day or two. But everything concerned with human life and fulfillment is nonexistent. The human being can't walk, can't speak, can't sing, can't whistle, and can't do anything. In fact, he can't do mathematics, can't do music; whatever you think, he can't do. Yet all these things will come to him. How? He has a highly developed nervous system. That nervous system has only one quality which is innate: curiosity. That curiosity is innate in all animals; otherwise, they wouldn't know where to go home and they wouldn't know how to avoid danger. The only real quality that is innate in human beings is curiosity. With that curiosity one will learn to realize what time is, what rhythm is, what singing means, what music means, what speaking means, walking, running, jumping, swimming—I don't know all the functions that a human being can do—functions which are all learned. There is such an amount of learning, and nobody knows how we learn to speak and nobody really knows how we come to learn to crawl and walk. By the time we deal with human beings, people like Piaget or General Smuts or anybody else, we deal with grown-up people; we believe that that's a human as he is. In fact, there isn't one of these systems that has not undergone an extraordinarily long period of organic learning, which is completely different from academic learning.

Academic learning has nothing to do with your personal growth unless by chance, occasionally. Therefore, it is not linked with time at all. It's a social event and a social necessity. We learn architecture because architecture is needed. We learn archeology, we learn engineering, we learn chemistry and computer science because society cannot exist without them, or exists better when it has those things. But none of them depend on or are linked with time in any way. I know Dr. Trager[2] was long ago something else and then he became a doctor; he could have not done it at all. He could have postponed it another fifty years. He could have taken it fifty years ago. It is not written that you should do medicine at all. I have not done medicine, though I wanted to, and I've never been to medical school. So you see, you can do whatever you like. You can stop it, you can postpone it; you can never do it, or do it at any chosen moment of your life. But try to skate before you can walk! Can you? Try to walk before you have crawled. Anybody who has begun by walking without crawling already has defects and will need Dr. Trager or somebody else to help him. When you think of that, we can begin to see that fulfillment is not just a simple thing, provided we think of how a baby becomes a human being, a grown-up human being. You will find that there is a period of organic learning where you cannot alter the time, the sequence, or the length of it. You have practically no say. In academic learning you are the master; it's a social thing.

Let's go back to fulfillment. See the learned things we have done: to speak, to walk, to stand, to write, to read, to make music, and to understand and deal with mathematics. You can see most of our occupations and in these find life fulfillment or self-fulfillment is a necessity. Suppose you can't walk. You grew up and you can't walk. You might have cerebral palsy, dystonia, muscular dystrophy; you might have God knows what. There are hundreds of diseases which will interfere with your walking. Life fulfillment for you or for me may be to be able to walk, or to be able to stand without support, or move without a wheelchair. That's a fulfillment. If I can't speak, if I stutter, it may be a life fulfillment to be able to speak clearly. Some people may have a life's fulfillment in singing. For instance, singing and music were eliminated from my childhood by my father's attitude of being a learned man. He thought it was futile to whistle or sing. I should deal with mathematics, with learning—which I did, of course. At the age of seventy I gave myself a birthday present, because up to seventy I had received about two hundred neckties for birthday presents, and I don't wear neckties anymore. The first present I gave to myself was two years of learning to play the piano. My teacher was a pupil of mine, a composer named Lockner. Then I learned singing for three years. Only then, by doing that when I was already seventy-five, did I realize what I had missed all my life. I regret today that I did not start when I was fifteen, or twelve. So you see, it's in all those things we learn that there is a question of fulfillment. There's a question of fulfillment if you can't walk; it's a fulfillment to be able to walk. If you have cerebral palsy with athetosis it may be a fulfillment to be more or less like everyone else—which is never the same thing as being yourself. You find that in these limitations in organic learning there is a question of fulfillment.

Now let's see further. Singing, music, mathematics, whistling, walking, swimming—all the actions that are possible, and the elimination of all the troubles that can happen to a human being—may be life fulfillment. I have some extraordinary examples of somebody fulfilling his life. I define health in a funny sort of way I'm sure none of you do. When I say I'm sure, maybe I am wrong, because the unexpected always happens. I have, I believe, a few original ways of looking at health, not because I tend to be original, but because I am doing things in a concrete way. And you can see how concrete it is; my first definition of health is somebody who is capable of realizing his or her unavowed dreams. Believe it or not, most people had intentions of organizing their lives when they were children or when they were adolescents that were stamped out of them in the long run. But these unavowed dreams remained active in them so they can be miserable all their lives having everything they want, but still being dissatisfied, feeling that their life was not fulfilled. For instance, somebody wants to paint, feels that he or she is a painter, and all her life has no chance. Conditions are such that it is impossible. I have an example of that in my own mother. My mother began to paint at eighty, but until eighty she didn't have a minute when she could do it. She painted until ninety-three and produced a series of pictures that many painters admire. There are unavowed dreams in many people; in fact, in every one of us. Salvador Dali—I don't know whether you read his biography—said that when he was five years old he wanted to be a fireman. A year later he decided he wanted to be Napoleon. Since then, his ambitions keep on growing. So you see, there are many examples like that.

Having defined health as I told you, I had an extraordinary occasion in New York City only a few weeks ago. I gave a workshop in New York at the Statler Hilton. There were 350 people, and it was a week's work. Among them were some crippled people; several were in wheelchairs and one woman came in with two four-pronged walkers. I couldn't understand why she came, what she wanted to get from my *Awareness Through Movement* lessons, how she would improve—but usually they do. People helped her to lie down on the floor and helped her to get up. Then at one moment people said, "You teach us *Awareness Through Movement*. We have heard of *Functional Integration* (which is individual nonverbal contact with a person). Would you show us what it is? We would like to understand and to have a concrete experience of it." I said, "All right." I looked around and said, "Is there one here who is really crippled?" Because if I do only a half-hour's work and the person is not really crippled, when he gets up you won't know whether he has been hypnotized, or exactly what happened by my shaking him here or there. I wanted something where there was nothing that could make that person different enough in an hour or so. I looked around, and picked this woman. She has cerebral palsy and is forty-nine years old. She is an intelligent woman, like many cerebral palsy people are. She is the librarian of the La Rochelle Library in New York. I told her to come with me, we improvised a table, and I put her on the table. I told them I would work on her about five minutes, not saying a word, so that she would not be influenced by what I said. Then I would repeat to them in words the same things, in the order I did them, so they could understand what I had done. First, the order is important, the number of movements you do, and all sorts of things. I worked on the woman and it turned out, with speaking, it took much longer than I expected. It took about three-quarters of an hour. When we finished, she was crying and laughing at the same time. A hundred people in the audience literally wept seeing the difference that took place. I took the woman off the table, took one hand, with her in a dancing position, and said, "You just follow what you feel. Do nothing." I moved her very gently and in a minute or so we were waltzing, she was waltzing. Then she left, forgetting the walkers near the table. Later she came to Amherst, where we train our 235 new Practitioners to increase the numbers in the *Feldenkrais* GUILD. She carried one walker in her hand, literally, carried it, and then came and stood while I presented her to the audience. She put the walker aside and stood the whole day on her feet. She said, "That was an unavowed dream: to be able to stand." In New York, she actually told me, "Now that this unavowed dream is realized, give me another dream."

In other words, when we talk about fulfillment or self-fulfillment, you can see that the thing is actually much more complex than just, say, self-fulfillment. If you have a concrete way of seeing it, you have concrete ways of helping. You cannot have concrete ways unless you know how we grow from a baby who can't speak, can't walk, can't do whistling, singing, speaking, mathematics, times, and rhythms, doesn't know anything, and learns all these things. How does a baby come to the state we are in? Obviously all these things cannot be taught to every child because it is the child who learns. *You* can't teach him what you want. *He* learns and his way of learning is actually a sensory-motor way. The first year and a half it is done without thinking. Only if we understand how that growth, that initial

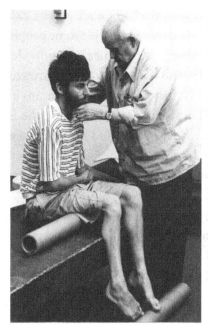
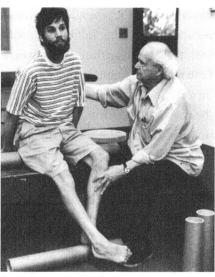
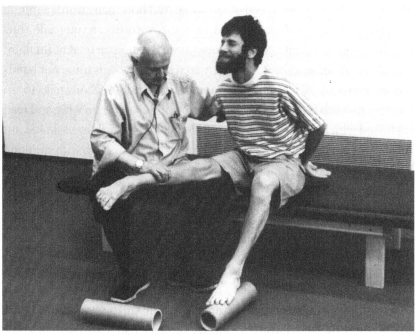

Feldenkrais working with Neil Marcus, 1981.

motor-sensory learning, becomes what we are when we are grown, can we understand what fulfillment means. Then we can provide some people with the means, within themselves, because I have no means to provide. I can make conditions in which they can learn to realize what their unavowed dream is, actually delve into it and find that they achieve also the means in themselves to perform it, to realize it. There is not a healthy person who is not like that. I believe that the person who never avowed his unavowed dreams somewhere in his unconscious, in his dreams, feels he has wasted his life, and when he is old he will realize it. So self-fulfillment is a real, vital necessity.

Once we come to organic learning you find, if you look at it from the same point of view—how the learning occurred and what it did to the person, how it is performed, and what learning means—it is absolutely different from what we usually think and it works in an extraordinary way. I can show you here and now some things which will probably make you wonder why you didn't think of them yourself—and you could. What is the speed of reading? It's the speed of speaking. And how many words a minute can you speak? About three hundred. How many words can you read? Three hundred words a minute. Now this looks as if it is a human quality. Bunkum. It isn't. It isn't because the way we learn to read and write is using our hands. You have to copy "A" a hundred thousand times and somebody talks to you and says that this is an "A." It takes you some time to learn to write and read. It's linked with hearing the words, pronouncing the words even slower, and the movement of the hands, which was done in conjunction with speaking. Therefore, it is linked. Our reading is linked with the rate of speaking, with the rate of writing. It's so wired-in in our nervous system because our nervous system learns to do things. It doesn't happen to the nervous system; it doesn't come out of the blue. It took years before we could read and write and speak. They are all linked together and the speed is set by the habit of the learning process. But these habits are completely divorced from our biological, physiological ability.

Everybody knows that there are now people in America who have learned to read three thousand words a minute; Kennedy could do that. There's no city in America, I think, where there are not speed-reading lessons. What do they do? A kind of thing I have been doing since 1947; I didn't know it was called speed-reading. I called it just becoming normal. The thing was divorcing speaking from thinking. This means learning not to use the speaking system, which is common to everybody and limits everybody. If you think in images, in patterns, if you are thinking visually, auditorially, with your smell, or kinesthetically, and you do not pronounce the words even subliminally, every one of you can learn in a few minutes to double the speed of reading, and of hearing also. By divorcing speaking from thinking, you are capable of reading with your eyes practically two or three lines in one look. People have learned to read at ten times the normal speed, or three thousand words a minute. They see the content clearer; therefore, retention is better and comprehension is better. I've seen a person reading a book like that, a chap called Dr. Frank. I gave him a book to read, and he turned the pages at ten seconds per page. I said, "What are you doing?" He said, "I'm reading the book." "Have you read it?" He said, "Yeah." "What is in it?" He told me everything in it. He had learned by doing it himself. Try it at home, and you will be surprised. Take a page and move across the first line with your hand, without trying to read it—just the first line, five, six times. Then a little slower, and a little faster, and you'll be surprised to find that suddenly you know what is written in that line. It's enough to do about ten or fifteen movements like that. You do it without having pronounced the words, and you know what is written in the line. Then do it with the second line; it goes faster, and the third line, still faster. You will find that if you spend a quarter of an hour on the first page just moving your hand across without trying to read, just looking, following your hand, you can read at the speed of moving your hand.

Once you have learned to divorce or separate speaking from seeing, not only can you read without pronouncing the words, and do it ten times faster than before, you discover your thinking was nil before that. When you think the way you are thinking now as you listen to me, what are you doing? The words are connected with what? When you speak now, what's connected to it? It is syntactically formed. It's formed in phrases. Which poet, painter, inventor, creator, has ever thought in syntax-formed language in his mind? It's impossible, because the thing he is doing, the thing he has created, is nonexistent. Therefore, there are no words for it, no phrase; there couldn't be syntax for it. In fact, you have to create a new word to express it, like Freud with the unconscious, or some mathematicians with imaginary numbers. How could you do mathematics with words? The way I'm talking now I can only say things that I have already thought at some earlier stage of my life, things I have read, things I have learned, things I have dreamed, and things other people told me. But none of that has to do with fulfillment of my life because I am actually acting out of memory, reliving, rehashing things that were done before. What sort of thinking is that? How would you think something new, creative? It may happen for only two seconds in your life, if at all. If you read the *Los Angeles Times,* the *New York Times,* the *Financial News* of Great Britain, and the *London Times* for twenty-five years, what will you be able to do after twenty-five years of reading? What has it improved in you?

The way I teach my students to work is to bring them into conditions where they can learn to think. They have to learn to think without words, with images, patterns, and connections. That sort of thinking always leads to a new way of action. With the gibberish talking and thinking we do now, we can talk for a donkey's age and nothing has changed. But if you think for one second in the way which eliminates the connection with words, you cannot think but in patterns, in disciplines connected to one another. You can't think otherwise than Edison, or Gauss, or Laplace.[3] You are thinking with the elements of thinking. Maybe whatever you do has already been invented by somebody, but you have invented it yourself. You have created it. So you can see, by learning speed-reading—divorcing or separating talking from thinking—you actually begin to think for the first time in your life, originally, creatively. You will be surprised what you can do. I was surprised.

I worked all my life as a physicist. I was with Joliot-Curie[4] for ten years. I was in the British Admiralty as a scientist, and many other places. Until the age of fifty I was a scientist. Since then, having come across the ideas I'm explaining to you now, I have created more than ten thousand recorded hours of human movement, two combinations of human movements. Only people who have been in contact with me will be able to do them. They are simple movements with the mouth and the hands, which are the most conscious parts of ourselves. I have created about ten thousand hours and recorded thirty variations in each one. In other words, I have composed more music than Beethoven and Bach together. Now I had no idea of that at all.

Now to give you a simple example: just extend your right arm in front of you, and twist the arm around until your palm faces to your right. Now cross your left arm over your right arm and interlace the fingers of your left hand with your right. Bring your interlaced hands toward you. Now go on, put your head into the hole formed by your arms. That's your habitual way of interlacing your fingers. What about doing the opposite, the nonhabitual one? People don't even know that they are able to do it. If you believe this is simple, I can assure you it is not. If you do the habitual one behind your head, you find it comfortable. You do the nonhabitual behind you, and you find that something is funny in the space around you. Obviously, it should be because if you exaggerate it you see what your system has learned. If I do the habitual interlacing of the hands, that hand, that shoulder and this hand and the head, do that. If I want to do it the other way around there must be a significant reorientation of the head and the eyes and the spine. If you lie down on the floor you will be surprised how different it is because the shoulder blades and the chest and everything move differently. You can see how these are movements people have never learned.

What do we want a nervous system for? Humanity, until a few hundred years ago, didn't know there was a nervous system at all. If you don't know that there is one, probably you don't need it. I believe that is actually the essence of it. Does any animal know he has a nervous system? Can't a lion or a cheetah run better than any human being without knowing at all that it has a nervous system? How many people can tell where the nervous system is? What do you know about it? In which condition is it? You don't know; I don't know either. In fact, it turns out in the way of looking at learning and growing, a good nervous system is one which you don't know that you have. As soon as that nervous system gets faulty, and you find you want to touch y-y-y-y-our n-n-n-nose and you c-c-can't get it, then you are very interested in what the nervous system is. The nervous system is the most pre-

cious thing on this earth. If you take away the water, which is ninety percent of the brain, the brain tissue in itself is the most precious organization
on this earth. It is rarer in quantity than cobalt, uranium, or anything. There
is much less of it than any of the precious things on this earth. It is so precious that the God, or nature, or whoever created us, made sure that none
of us will have access to it and put it there, inside our safe. Nature, evolution, thinks we are much too silly. If we had a finger to put in it, it would
never work. [If] it doesn't work in some human being, and someone has to
go and open it and have a look at it, it is better for us that that doesn't happen.
In other words, a healthy nervous system is not like a nervous system the
way we think of it in the normal way of speaking about holism—it is much
more. Actually, General Smuts saw it in practically the same way I do. It is
an extraordinarily important, complex thing that there is much to know
about and use.

I told you about reading. I will show you something even more striking—hearing and music. We normally remember melodies. We can remember notes through that technique of melody, and we can remember a lot of
single notes sung. We are used to reading and speaking at three hundred
words a minute. If I take a tape recorder and present you with what you
have heard, obviously you could hear it. I advise you to take a tape recorder
at home, at the normal rate it speaks, rewind that phrase, and press the fast-
forward button. You will be surprised that with the speed doubled you can
understand every word of the phrase you have already heard. Then rewind
two phrases, the one before that you never really heard, and you will find
you can hear the other one at double the speed. I assure you, take that tape
recorder and deal with it for ten minutes and you will learn to listen to and
understand every word. It doesn't matter if you are one hundred years old,
or twenty. This shows you what happens when you understand and inquire
into the human brain, as we do in *Functional Integration*. . . .

. . . we never use more than about ten percent of our abilities, except in
the one thing on which we build our life. There we use our full ability, or
almost all of it. But there is no reason why you shouldn't do this on every
level of your existence.

I hope you can realize all your unavowed dreams.

PART 2

Interviews

8

Image, Movement, and Actor: Restoration of Potentiality

Interview with Richard Schechner and Helen Schechner

Translated and edited by Kelly Morris

Richard Schechner is a well-known director, teacher, and author: he is a professor at the Tisch School of the Arts, New York University; editor of *TDR: The Drama Review;* and an active theater director. He is perhaps best known for his numerous books and articles concerning Performance Theory, which have been translated extensively and have an international readership.

Kelly Morris was a graduate student in the Department of Theatre at Tulane University at the time of this interview. The interview was conducted in English; however, Morris translated some text from an article in French, which he includes with the interview.*−Ed.*

This exposition of Feldenkrais's ideas and techniques of movement training is taken from two of his essays, "L'expression corporelle" and "Mind and Body." This material is interspersed with selections from an interview with Feldenkrais by Richard and Helen Schechner in Tel Aviv during June 1965.

Feldenkrais uses "body image" and "self-image" interchangeably; he claims that there is no valid distinction to be made between the "self" and the "mind-body." I have followed his not-quite-arbitrary usage. This exposition suffers, no doubt, from brevity. No attempt has been made to offer the available (and substantial) supporting demonstrations, argumentation, and data. Feldenkrais's concerns and practice are clearly applicable to theater training; and, although he does not allude to it here, he has worked with the Habima Theatre in Israel.—KM

Mind-Body Unity

FELDENKRAIS: My fundamental contention is that the unity of mind and body is an objective reality, that these entities are not related to each other in one fashion or another, but are an inseparable whole. To put this more clearly: I contend that a brain could not think without motor functions. It is probably language's serial formation in time which determines the serial genesis of our thoughts. Let me substantiate this: (1) It takes longer to think the numbers from twenty to thirty than from one to ten although the numerical intervals are the same for each series. The differences lie in the fact that the time intervals are proportional to the time needed to utter the corresponding numbers aloud. This suggests that we actually mobilize the vocal apparatus. Thus, one of the purest abstractions is inextricably linked with muscular activity. Most people cannot think clearly without mobilizing the motor function of the brain enough to become aware of the word patterns representing the thought. (2) Macular vision—distinct, clear seeing—is limited to a very small area at a time. To perceive clearly the content of what we see while reading takes us the time required for the muscles of the eyes to scan the area under inspection. Here again, we see the functional unity of perception and motor function. (3) Consider feeling in detail. I may feel joyful, angry, afraid, disgusted. Everyone can, on seeing me, recognize the feeling I experience. Which comes first: the motor pattern or the feeling? I would like to stress the idea that they are basically the same thing. We cannot become conscious of a feeling before it is expressed by a motor mobilization, and therefore *there is no feeling so long as there is no body attitude.*

SCHECHNER: The idea of duality is so deeply inbred into theater and into acting that it is difficult to uproot it. I wonder if you could explain the basis for your belief in the unity, and its sources and consequences.

94

FELDENKRAIS: Oh, it's a very, very long story. I have ten lectures on that, showing that we have no real basis for thinking of the duality except the habit of thought. You have never yet had an analysis made on the subconscious or the conscious without having the body brought to you. You cannot make a successful analysis without changing the expression of the face; that means it has something to do with the muscles.

SCHECHNER: But the duality-people say that there is a *relationship* but not an identity.

FELDENKRAIS: I also say that there is no identity. I say there is only one thing. There is a functioning of the nervous system inside, and that functioning has two aspects. If you listen to someone, you see the motor aspect and also perceive the mental aspect (the content of his words). Let us repeat that the state of the cortex is directly and legibly visible on the periphery through the attitude, posture, and muscular configuration, which are all connected. Any change in the nervous system translates itself clearly through a change of attitude, posture, and muscular configuration. They are not two states but two aspects of the same state.

SCHECHNER: How did you come upon your technique?

FELDENKRAIS: I played soccer in my young days, and I tore a cross ligament. Later it turned out that in the difficult moments of my life, during the German invasion of France and so on, the knee started troubling me and every second day the knee swelled; I couldn't walk. After a few years I went to see a surgeon. He examined the knee, took X-rays, and said, "Look, you need an operation. You can't go on like that." I asked, "Is there any likelihood that the operation will not be successful?" He said, "Oh, yes, it's about fifty-fifty." So I said, "Goodbye, I won't do it." He said, "You can't go on with that knee."

SCHECHNER: What did you do?

FELDENKRAIS: Before I had trouble with the knee I had had thirty years' experience with it. I spent a lot of time using the knee properly, but eventually I forgot that old, good way.

SCHECHNER: So you very carefully reconstructed your movements?

FELDENKRAIS: Yes, it was a real discovery. I found out that I was holding the ground, that I was afraid of slipping with the knee. I was actually making it slip, but I didn't realize it. I began using the knee correctly and I found it easier.

SCHECHNER: And that started you on the idea of body image?

FELDENKRAIS: No, I didn't think of body image in the beginning.

SCHECHNER: How did you come around to that idea?

FELDENKRAIS: Well, after the knee was all right, I slipped on a banana skin and the whole thing was undone. That gave me a shock, because until that time I thought I was doing only what I had decided to do. Here I discovered that at the moment of the fall I forgot about my theory and did the wrong thing. I slipped like any normal person would. It was new to me that things were happening in me in spite of my own awareness, in spite of my own decision. I realized that I was moving without knowing what I was doing. I acted myself in a crisis. I then saw that most people don't know what they are doing; they just don't know that they don't know. So I read a lot of physiology and psychology and to my great astonishment I found that in regard to using the whole human being for action, there was ignorance, superstition, and absolute idiocy. There wasn't a single book that dealt with *how* we function.

The Self-Image and Reality

FELDENKRAIS: Each person has an impression of his own manner of speaking, walking, and carriage which seems personal and immutable—the only possible way—and he identifies himself with this image. His judgment of the spatial relationships and movements of his body seems innate, and he believes it is possible to change only the vitality, intensity, and capability of them. But everything important for social relations is acquired through a long apprenticeship: one learns to walk, to speak, to see the third dimension in a painting or photograph. It is by the chance circumstances of birthplace and environment that one acquires specific movements, attitudes, language, etc. The difficulty in changing a physical or mental habit is due partly to heredity and individuality, but mostly to the necessity of displacing an already-acquired habit.

It would be well at this point to perform a simple exercise, so that one may actually feel the conditions and possibilities I am describing. Lie down on your back; mentally and methodically scan your entire body. You will discover that you can concentrate on certain parts more easily than others, and that you usually lose consciousness of these other parts during an action. In fact, certain parts almost never figure in the self-image during action.

For example, close your eyes and try to represent the width of your mouth with your index fingers. It is not unusual to discover an error of up to three hundred percent in exaggeration or underestimation. Keeping your eyes closed, try to represent with your hands the thickness of your chest, first with your hands in back and front, then by separating them laterally, and finally vertically. You will be amazed to see that your judgment changed with the positions of your hands and that for each attempt you produced a different result. The variation is often as much as one hundred percent.

When this deviation between the conception of the self-image and the objective (or "real") facts is nearly one hundred percent, the behavior of that part of the body is generally defective. For example: Someone who holds his chest in a position of exaggerated exhalation will find that according to his self-image the chest seems two or three times thicker than it is in reality. Inversely, someone who holds a position of extreme inhalation will find the self-image underestimates the chest's thickness. A detailed examination of the whole body—particularly the pelvic and genital-anal region—will reveal even greater surprises.

If one simply thinks of his accustomed manner as an alternate term for "self-image," one comprehends the difficulty in perfecting a particular action. The self-image's habitual configuration is to a certain extent compulsive; the person could not act otherwise. He substitutes a habitual action for the proposed exercise without being conscious of not doing what he wished.

The difficulty, therefore, is not bound up with the substance of the habit, but with the temporal order—that is, the priority of the formed pattern that, in itself, is simply a product of chance. The question, then, is: Is it possible to so change the body-attitude that new manners, different by choice, would be as fully personal as those previously acquired, without taking into account the person's past life? It is important to understand that I do not intend the simple substitution of one action for another (which would be "static"), but a change in the mode of action, achieved through the "dynamic" of activity in general.

Movement and Posture

FELDENKRAIS: Can *you* define good movement?

SCHECHNER: No, except on stage I would say good movement is that which suits the part; but it's easier to recognize bad movement than to say what's good about good movement.

FELDENKRAIS: Yes, but when you say it should suit the part, you're not offering a definition, and you couldn't teach people good movement with a loose notion of what it is.

SCHECHNER: What is good movement?

FELDENKRAIS: Well, good movement is more complex than it seems. First of all, it should be reversible. For instance, if I make a movement with my hand it will be accepted as good, as conscious, clear, and willed movement if I can at any point of the trajectory stop, reverse the movement, continue, or change it into something else.

SCHECHNER: And you think that a basic definition of acting is the reversibility of the gesture?

FELDENKRAIS: Not only the gesture but the whole attitude. The actor should be able to stop, start again, or do something else. Only then can he play ten nights, one after the other, and do the same thing. Reversibility is one part of it. The next important thing is that the body should be maintained in a state of action where it can start a movement without preliminaries. For instance, suppose I normally stand with my feet wide apart. I have stability this way, but can't walk without first shifting around completely. Though this is the "best" posture by definition, I cannot move forward or backwards. This is the extreme case of *bad* posture. Now if I stand with a leg forward and back bent, I can of course walk forward or backwards. But if somebody asked me to jump, I couldn't do it without changing my position. But if I stand so that I can, without preliminaries, rise, stoop, move forward, backwards, right and left, and twist myself—then elementary demands of good posture are fulfilled. This is also true for the voice and the breath.

SCHECHNER: So when you talk about movement, you're working with the voice, the breath, the movement, the eyes, the ears—the total body organism. You must be working with the total mental organism too.

FELDENKRAIS: Absolutely! They are one. I am working with the *human* organism.

Consciousness and Rebirth Through Reversibility

SCHECHNER: Is awareness implicit in reversibility?

FELDENKRAIS: Yes. Of course, when you are fully aware of a movement you can change the intensity, speed, rhythm, and intonation. An act can be reflective, unconscious, automatic, or fully conscious and aware. Acquiring a new mode of doing needs awareness ontogenetically or individually. When

learning is completed the action may become automatic or even unconscious. Phylogenetically learned action is reflective. Thus "consciousness,"
or "awareness," has no meaning except as a description or qualification of
activity.

SCHECHNER: How is this awareness related to body image?

FELDENKRAIS: An actor who doesn't feel his changes of position relative
to partners has no real spatial awareness—he can never reply. He waits for
the other actor to stop and then he says his part.

SCHECHNER: The actor who is performing a role is in a different relationship to his body image than a person in everyday life. He's enacting someone else's body image. And in a sense he has to know about it beforehand,
and yet it has to seem spontaneous. I wonder if I could ask you specifically
how this work would help an actor who is playing Don Juan or Hamlet?

FELDENKRAIS: He must be trained to have the fluent ability to act and
check what that action means in reality. He should be able to act not only
Hamlet, but even a woman.

SCHECHNER: Why does awareness increase the ability of an actor to relate
to another actor?

FELDENKRAIS: It helps the actor listen to the other person.

SCHECHNER: How do you go about teaching this awareness?

FELDENKRAIS: Our first awareness of the outside world is through the
mouth. Most people are aware of their mouths, lips, and tongues more than
of any other parts of the body. The awareness of the rest of the body in our
culture is a matter of chance. For instance, some people are completely
unaware of their ears and their hearing. The trouble is not so much that
they do not hear, but that they are not aware of the relation of the ear to the

mouth, of hearing to speaking. Thus, when they hear their voice recorded for the first time they are completely staggered, because they never listen to themselves.

The crucial work consists in leading to awareness in *action,* or the ability to make contact with one's own skeleton and muscles and with the environment nearly simultaneously. This is not relaxation, for true relaxation can be maintained only when doing nothing. The aim is healthy, powerful, easy, and pleasurable exertion (eutony).* The reduction of tension is necessary because efficient movement is effortless. Inefficiency is sensed as effort and prevents one doing more and better.

The gradual reduction of useless effort is necessary in order to increase kinetic sensitivity, without which a person cannot become self-regulating. The Fechner-Weber law shows clearly that for a certain range of human sensations and activities the difference in stimulus (I) that produces the least detectable difference in sensation (S) is always in the same ratio to the whole stimulus: Change in $S = K$ (change in I/I) or $S = \text{Log } I + \text{Constant}$.**

To explain it in simple terms, if you carry a piano on your back, and a fly lands on the piano, you will not be able to feel any additional weight. But if a big dog sat there you might notice. Now the question is: What is the amount that you have to add or subtract to notice it?

SCHECHNER: The proportion will always be the same.

FELDENKRAIS: Yes, for the kinesthetic sensation, the feeling of weight, it's about a fortieth. So you see, if you want to perceive the difference (feel the fly), you must reduce the amount of stimulus present (and carry something

---

Eutony comes from Greek and could be translated as "balanced tonus." Gerda Alexander (1908–1994) called her somatic approach to self-development "Eutony," which she taught in Denmark. She described it as "tonicity in constant adaptation to the state or activity of the moment," much as Feldenkrais is using it here and later in the interview. Feldenkrais knew Gerda Alexander well. The two approaches share many similarities and Feldenkrais is clearly taking inspiration from Alexander here in his use of the term *eutony.*

**For more about the Weber-Fechner law see the discussion on pages xvi–xvii and the footnote on page 37.—*Ed.*

rather lighter than a piano). That's why I get the students down on the floor. Unless the necessary muscular tension is reduced, they couldn't detect any changes.

If you perform a careful examination—exercise with the head, dipping, raising, and turning it slowly, focusing attention on spatial orientation and the relationships between the different parts of the left side (the head with the left shoulder, the collarbone, the spine, etc.)—you will find an equal change of latent tone on the whole left side. These important conclusions may be drawn: (1) When the two sides participate symmetrically in the movements of lowering and raising the head, the tonic change, the feeling of well-being, and the ease of control gained are experienced *only on the side where the spatial relations are clear and conscious.* Both sides participate equally, but only one side benefits from the movement. (2) The change is produced somewhere in the central nervous system, for one whole side was affected—exclusively the side on which we worked. (3) The change does not disappear instantly, but can last several hours or several days, depending above all on the clarity of conception of the spatial relationships and the mnemonic retention of the difference between the two sides.

The importance of what has happened in the nervous system is accentuated by the fact that *one can produce the same effect in the other side by predominantly mental work.* While the first effect was obtained in a half-hour or hour, methodical concentration on differences in kinesthetic sensations in the two sides—from the toes to the top of the head—takes only two or three minutes and is completed when equalization of sensation is experienced. Perhaps the most important point is that however satisfied one might have been with the habitual carriage of his head or foot when beginning the exercise, the work produces a contrast which compels one to appreciate how far habitual self-management is from what it *could be.*

By judicious selection and appropriate exercises, one eventually eliminates the habitual restrictions on possible configurations in action. Mechanical repetition of an action is not a valuable step in image expansion and exploration; it is only a muscular exertion. In order for an exercise to produce the development and clarification of the self-image, it must include concentration on: (1) each part of the action itself, (2) what is felt during the action, (3) the total body image, and the effect of the action on the body image. Only with this constant surveillance and reassessment can one progress to new actions, orientations, and adjustments.

A careful application of the theory of reversibility produces these results: (1) the configuration and relationships of the skeleton are made conscious; (2) the latent tension of the whole muscle-structure is reduced and equalized; (3) reduction of effort in all areas of activity; (4) simplification of movement and therefore facilitation of all action; (5) improvement of the power of orientation; (6) reduction of fatigue and therefore greater capacity for work and perseverance; (7) improvement of posture and breathing, and therefore an improvement of general health and vigor; (8) improvement of coordination in all actions; (9) facilitation of learning in all areas, physical or mental; (10) a more profound self-knowledge.

Eutony

FELDENKRAIS: Most people do not realize the amount of useless strain they have in their eyes, mouth, legs, stomachs. This strain is harmful, mostly because the keenness of our self-realization depends on the amount of strain that is present.

SCHECHNER: In other words, to really concentrate, the strain must be decreased. Doesn't this relate to some of Stanislavski's* theories of relaxation, that to concentrate one must first know how to relax?

FELDENKRAIS: But not just to relax, because if you really relax you can't do anything! A properly relaxed person has difficulty in collecting his members to move. What we want is eutony, which doesn't mean lack of tension, but directed and controlled tension with excessive strain eliminated. This

---

*Constantin Stanislavski (1863–1938) developed a naturalistic approach to training actors that has been highly influential throughout the international theater world. He stressed the importance of psychophysical training and relaxation in the education of an actor, stating that "muscular tautness interferes with inner emotional experience."

is not flaccidity, but muscular tension only equivalent to the demands of gravity.

SCHECHNER: And how do you train to get this perfect balance?

FELDENKRAIS: We have an inexhaustible series of techniques. First, very small movement. If you lie down and try to lift your head, say, one-hundredth of an inch, and lower it again, and do that quickly thirty or forty times, and then stop, you'll find an incredibly heightened awareness of what's happening there. Stand flat-footed, and then raise your heels and let your body drop back. Fifty small movements like that and you'll suddenly detect incorrect standing. Go on, do it. Now try to walk. What do you feel? A coming down?

SCHECHNER: It's really weird. Much lighter.

FELDENKRAIS: Some people have one leg shorter than the other, and they never discover it until they do that. Then they suddenly discover which is the shorter leg and what they can do about it. If you press and stiffen your spine thirty seconds or so, and then let go, you'll see that it changes your posture more than a month's training. This is accomplished by changing relationships of muscles throughout the spine.

SCHECHNER: Then you finally learn how to do these things without physical stimulus?

FELDENKRAIS: Oh, yes. You can reinstate the same organization in yourself without doing anything.

SCHECHNER: Suppose an actor learns to develop his consciousness, his sense of his self-image. There is the feeling among actors that if they lose their spontaneity, they lose their art.

FELDENKRAIS: If you look at it properly, what we mean by spontaneity is just to be an idiot. How on earth can an actor be spontaneous?

SCHECHNER: Well, they want to maintain "the illusion of the first time." They want to feel what they call free.

FELDENKRAIS: But they can't do it if they're not aware of what they're doing, and those actors who claim to do it give an abysmal performance on one day and a perfect one on the next.

SCHECHNER: Are you aware of Lee Strasberg's* work?

FELDENKRAIS: Oh, yes.

SCHECHNER: Well?

FELDENKRAIS: Strasberg wanted me to teach. He said he would open a school for acting in Israel if I was willing to be a teacher there. I came to the Actors Studio and he presented me to all the people there and we talked about it very favorably.

SCHECHNER: How long ago was that?

FELDENKRAIS: Four years ago.

SCHECHNER: Nothing came of it?

FELDENKRAIS: Nothing.

SCHECHNER: But of course the work that he does at the Studio seems contrary to the kind of work that you do.

FELDENKRAIS: I saw the work of the Studio many times. I liked it. I don't think it's ideal from my point of view, but Strasberg's method interested me.

---

*Lee Strasberg (1901–1982) was one of the developers of "Method acting" and founded the Actors Studio in New York, a prestigious and influential acting school. In Method acting the actors draw on their own emotions and memories to portray a character.

SCHECHNER: It hasn't produced, in the United States at least, a dependable style of acting. An actor can be very good one night and very bad the next. It surprises me that you like Strasberg, because he's working toward a lack of consciousness rather than consciousness.

FELDENKRAIS: I am a funny person. I like the work, but that doesn't mean that I agree with it. His whole technique is deficient, and I believe that if he corrected it from my point of view he would get much better results. You see, his is a limited demand on the actor. But when the actor is well trained, aware of his body, his mouth, his eyes, his volitions, and has full contact between the outside and the inside, he can pick his own way.

SCHECHNER: What you're doing is basic human training.

FELDENKRAIS: Yes. You have a cortex, some parts of which are at all times mobilized. It is this constant stimulus that must be reduced. The Fechner-Weber law is true for sound, for light, for odor, for touch, for anything. The index for light is about one in one hundred eighty; for hearing, one in two hundred. That means that if you lit one hundred light bulbs and put one out you could be aware of it. But if there were one thousand bulbs, you'd never miss the one. So, to balance the cortex means to reduce all points of excitation to normal activity. In this pursuit, you will find that there is no point of excitation possible without an inhibition. In reducing the excitation, you also relieve the inhibition. When you level the cortex, you bring it to that state which some people call nirvana and we call eutony. Suddenly your brain becomes quiet and you see things that you never saw before. The possibility of making new combinations, which were inhibited before, is restored. The great value of this technique is that by reducing tension in a particular group of muscles, it provides a methodical study of the entire self-image, and through study, improvement. The technique shows clearly that the faults in self-organization are due to arrested self-development. The correction of these flaws is neither conceived nor experienced as the treatment of a disease but as a general *resumption of growth and development on all levels.*

SCHECHNER: And these combinations will be as legitimate and as real as the old ones?

FELDENKRAIS: Yes, perhaps more so. You discover, rediscover yourself as your structure is capable of being yourself to the limits of your body. You can be reborn.

Restoration of Potentiality

Generalized and improved behavior of the skeleton results in the full exploitation of anatomical possibilities. Most often, the limitation that one imputes to a lack of suppleness is actually due to the contraction and shortening of muscles through habit and lack of conscious appreciation. These habits produce deformations and unbalanced movement. The degeneration of skeletal articulation automatically enforces a new limitation on the muscles that then seek to avoid painful and uncomfortable movement. Thus the vicious circle begins, leading to a deformation of the skeleton, the spine, and the spinal disks; this makes the body prematurely aged, reducing the range and variety of movement. Experience shows us that age has only a minimal influence on such limitations, and that the ability to perform all movements allowed by skeletal and anatomical structure can be restored.

Reasonable, healthy people, free from serious disease, can achieve this remarkable state by an hour of work for each year of age, up to sixty years. Beyond that, intelligence and desire determine the amount of time.

SCHECHNER: There are exciting possibilities here, because the theater is the only art which demands the re-creation of human beings, I mean complete human beings.

FELDENKRAIS: Yes.

SCHECHNER: You said with some of these exercises that you come back to the basic human walk, and only the peculiarities of a person's walk distinguish it from another's. What would seem to happen with that training for an actor would be the arrival at a state of neutrality. Without this neutrality you are not conscious enough to take in the peculiarities of the character. So your idea is to achieve a kind of neutrality from which any direction is possible.

FELDENKRAIS: Yes, and you find that you can do it.

SCHECHNER: There are many explorations in terms of consciousness expansion and it seems that this is a much more systematic approach to the same business. Perhaps neutrality isn't the right word, but a broader consciousness that actually transforms rather than just brings the human being back to neutrality.

FELDENKRAIS: It is actually quite different from the idea of neutrality. That generality I am talking about is bringing the motor cortex, which has evolved without training, into an even state of excitation. Now if you take a normal cortex which has evolved without training, then out of the whole possibilities of the human body, out of the seventy languages that are possible, he has picked one. And where are all the other combinations? In the motor cortex we have fixed connections, patterns; and the wide range of possibilities that were there from before are circumscribed and cramped. You have linked them into fixed patterns and that's that.

SCHECHNER: So we're really talking about potentiality.

FELDENKRAIS: That's it exactly. I want the neutrality only to free you from the inhibition of having one specialty.

SCHECHNER: Now in terms of the normal everyday human being, this will allow him "to be more himself"?

FELDENKRAIS: Yes, sure.

SCHECHNER: This will allow the actor or dancer to assume whatever characteristics he wishes for the role?

FELDENKRAIS: Yes, with great clarity and ease. Today you can find an actor portraying a hunchback and talking like a gigolo, because he doesn't feel any connection. He wants a "nice" voice. Most actors, no matter what the role, speak the same way. If you record them and play them backwards you will hear the same rhythm, no matter what he says or what part he plays. And I find it boring.

SCHECHNER: Did you speak to Aharon Meskin* about what he meant when he said that Vakhtangov** and Stanislavski had the same intentions as you?

FELDENKRAIS: He said that he only now realizes the meaning of what they said. They often showed examples but could not teach what they wanted.

SCHECHNER: That was because they didn't have a systematic approach to it?

FELDENKRAIS: Because they had no body awareness themselves. They didn't know how to do it. If I start to tell you that the movement is wrong, I will convince you by rules, aspects, definitions that everybody will try. A hundred people, a thousand people will all agree that that is right and that is wrong. But with Stanislavski and others, if he said something was right or wrong it was only his own impression. He was right very often because he was a great man.

SCHECHNER: Are you going to work for a theater? It would be very interesting to see a generation of actors, ten or fifteen or twenty actors, fully trained in this technique.

---

*Aharon Meskin (1897–1974) was a well-known Israeli actor who worked in Israel and abroad. He acted often on Broadway in the '40s, '50s, and '60s. He and Moshe Feldenkrais were very close friends. Feldenkrais chose his home in Tel Aviv partly to live near Meskin.

**Yevgeny Bagrationovich Vakhtangov (1883–1922) was a legendary Russian theater director who used Stanislavski's techniques creatively, integrating them with other approaches.

FELDENKRAIS: You see, I am now involved in so many things that unless there is a demand from the outside . . .

* * *

I contacted Richard Schechner to ask him about his recollections of Feldenkrais and the interview. This is how he answered on April 10, 2010. –*Ed.*

I remember Moshe—and perhaps this memory is faulty—it is (I believe) from 1965, during my first trip to Israel. I remember Moshe as a "roly-poly" man, physically speaking: round and not tall, smiling and fast-talking, with an ebullience, confidence, and infectious optimism—about himself, about life.

He seemed to know everyone in Israel. I met Feldenkrais because I had long suffered from a "bad back," pains in my lower back that sometimes made it hard for me to walk. While in Israel, I had an attack. I was pretty much immobilized. Someone suggested I see Moshe Feldenkrais. "He can help you," I was told. "He knows everything about what is troubling you."

So I was taken to see him. We talked. He watched me walk. Then he suggested that I go down on my hands and feet, not my hands and knees, but my hands and feet, with my butt way up in the air. He told me to walk around on the floor that way, the way animals walk. "This will help you," he said. I recall that he spoke in English, but with a "European" accent, maybe German—but this placing of his accent as German (and not Hebrew) is probably due to my knowing that his name is "Feldenkrais," and that would place him as German-derived.

Anyway, I walked around the room for a few minutes as Moshe instructed. And—miraculously, it seemed to me—my pain was lessened, almost gone entirely. "You do this every morning when you get up," he said. And I did, and I have never had such a pain in my back again in my whole life. From time to time, I walk on my hands and feet the way animals do. But mostly I do not walk the way Feldenkrais taught me to anymore. In 1971 when I went to India for the first time, I studied yoga with Krishnamacharya, a great teacher. I still practice yoga. My back does not trouble me at all.

After meeting Moshe and his "fixing" my back, we began talking. I do not know whether it was after that meeting or after my interviewing him for *TDR* that we went together from Tel Aviv to Jerusalem. But I remember Moshe telling me, or asking me, if I wanted to go to Jerusalem with him. Or me telling him that I had to go to Jerusalem and he responding that he would take me or at least accompany me. And of course I said yes, I would love to go with him, or him with me: both of us together. I believe I had to go to Jerusalem for the meetings that brought me to Israel in the first place. I think it was a meeting of the International Theatre Institute (ITI).

When I asked Moshe how we would get from Tel Aviv to Jerusalem, he replied, "Let's walk." But, I said to him, "It's a long way." "Don't worry," he told me with happy confidence, giving me a big smile. So we went into the street and started to walk.

I will never forget what happened next. Every few minutes a car would pull over to the side of the road and someone would speak to Moshe. They knew him. I believe they were asking him if he wanted a lift somewhere. It seemed he was famous all over Israel, or at least in Tel Aviv, and he was also well known for his long walks. We walked and talked for a long time, maybe thirty or forty-five minutes or maybe even longer. Every so often a car would simply pull over and ask Moshe if he wanted a ride. Finally, he accepted a ride and we both got into the car and we were driven to Jerusalem. I was very impressed by how many people knew Moshe. And also by the sense of community, even family, I felt in Israel at that time.

I will say in some kind of conclusion that, somehow, at a very deep level, he and I hit it off. I was a young man of thirty-one years; I do not know how old he was at the time. But he seemed old and wise to me. And he helped me. And I felt a really strong connection with him. I still feel that forty-five years later ... he was sixty-one years old when we met ... about twice my age.

9

Feldenkrais Revisited: Tension, Talent, and the Legacy of Childhood

Interview with Joanna Rotté

Joanna Rotté, PhD, a professor of theater, conducted this interview in the early 1980s in Amherst, Massachusetts. It was published in 1998 in *New Theatre Quarterly*. Dr. Rotté is an active writer, actor, and director. She teaches script analysis and movement at Villanova University. *—Ed.*

A few years before he died, I interviewed Moshe Feldenkrais on the campus of Hampshire College in Amherst, Massachusetts, where he was conducting a nine-week teacher-training program in Feldenkrais methodology.... When I met Feldenkrais, his posture and carriage appeared comfortable. His shoulders looked relaxed. His gait was like a broom, kept close to the floor. He wore black cotton trousers in martial arts style and a blousy white, Indian-influenced shirt on a not tall but sturdy frame. On his feet were black Chinese-like cloth shoes. His own being modeled his intention: To restore each person to their human dignity.

I asked him to speak to his practice of getting at the mind through the body: Why this emphasis on using movement to teach the body to reprogram the brain?

EVERY ACTOR KNOWS THE ESSENTIALITY OF MOVEMENT. The important thing about movement is: Can he walk? Can he stand by himself? Can she go to the toilet by herself? Can she see to the right and the left? Can she hear? In other words, as far as movement goes, how can you imagine life without it? Obviously, it's the most general thing and the most important capacity for any person. A person who doesn't move at all—if he doesn't breathe and has no heartbeat, no regurgitating, and no defecation—surely he is dead.

Your teaching is addressed to the average person, to increase or heighten his or her awareness through movement. But the average person can already walk and stand and turn....

Oh, that's what he thinks!

... perhaps not well.

It's not a question of "well." I'm not interested in anybody walking well. I'm interested in him. A person comes to me and says, "My posture is bad," or he comes and says, "My breathing is bad." People come. I never ask them. I have never told anyone, "You have a bad posture and your eyes are cock-eyed and your head is tilted"; it's not my business.

So, the average person can believe that his posture is all right but can get to work, can improve their feeling about their posture. Your feeling, that's all. Your posture must change in such a way that it becomes to you a good feeling. Do you feel your breathing is as perfect as you want? Is your eyesight good?

My eyesight is not so good, but my breathing is all right.

Well, there you are. If you ask people, they'll say, "My voice is not so good." People complain. The average person complains. If the average person were feeling well, he wouldn't be doing any jogging. There are millions of people jogging in America. Why do they jog?

To feel better.

Because they feel bad. They feel they're clumsy. And, by the way, their jogging is not that good either. There are few people who jog and improve. So there is a question about jogging. Is your swimming perfect? Can you swim as well as Mark Spitz?

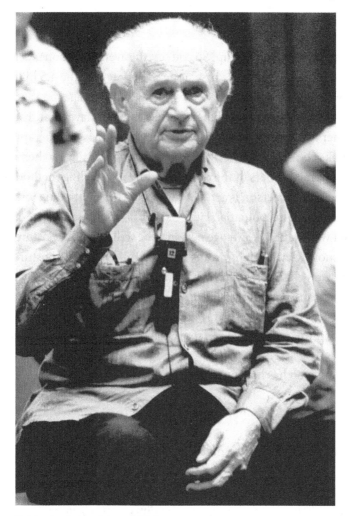

Feldenkrais teaching, 1981.

No.

Why not? You're an average person.

Insufficient training.

Training only? There are plenty of people who train to swim and none swims like Mark Spitz.

Insufficient desire.

The average person gives it up! So you see, the average person is actually the most interesting person, because none or very few of the 4.5 billion average people are satisfied with their own being. But average men and women are too silly to understand all their problems. They have their trouble, and they either just keep it to themselves or they go into psychotherapy. Or they read books about holistic health and try to do something by themselves, or they go to practitioners of the dozens of different healing methods taught.

So the average person is actually aware that he is not doing justice to his own makeup, to his potential. He feels that he could be better. So, you see, it is not I who wants the average person to be well, to get his posture straight. I don't know what straight means for him. If I make your posture the way I like it, you will find it awful. I must make your posture the way that feels to you to be the posture you'd like to feel.

Is that what you mean when you speak of a correct self-image for each person?

Yes, each person has his own makeup.

And the correct image cannot come from outside oneself?

No, it cannot. Because if it could, a person would have it.

Will there always be some conflict within a person between the society's image of what he should be and his own personally correct self-image?

In our society, in our culture, it is unavoidable. But some anthropologists have found a very few, very small communities in the world where it isn't like this. They haven't got the big problems of big countries where the solutions are not simple.

So your way for a person to reach his correct self-image is through action?

Yes, because without action we can't know what we would like to feel.

And you teach that one of the crucial factors contributing to a person's getting away from his correct self-image is the experience of pain.

Yes, most of the problems people have come through pain, whether it is tooth pain, eye pain, neck pain, ear pain, stomach pain.

Or social pain? Or pain from one's parents?

Yes, emotional pain—deep insults to a child, let us say, who loses all confidence and does not consider himself worthy of standing on his own feet.

But how do I know when I'm manifesting my correct self-image?

Actually, to say the word *correct* is not correct. Can you see? Knowing this in itself actually helps you already to understand that you are not going to be given a series of rules that you would have to hold your head like this, your hand like that, and your feet like this, and then you would be all right. That would be cuckoo, wouldn't it?

If I want to help you to feel comfortable in your mind, I must bring you to a state that you feel is correct for you. The state you are brought to must be one which makes you a more effective person with more direct performance of your intention. You must be helped to get to a state where you have a good nervous system, but do not need to know that you have a nervous system.

For example, if you want to take a good look at me, you take it. At this point, you don't need to know that you have a nervous system. You only need to focus and press a sight button. But if another person wants to take a good look at me and he has a tremor in his neck, then he knows that he has a tremor and a nervous system, and he would go to a neurologist to find out what's wrong with his nervous system. In other words, a well-organized nervous system is one you don't know you have.

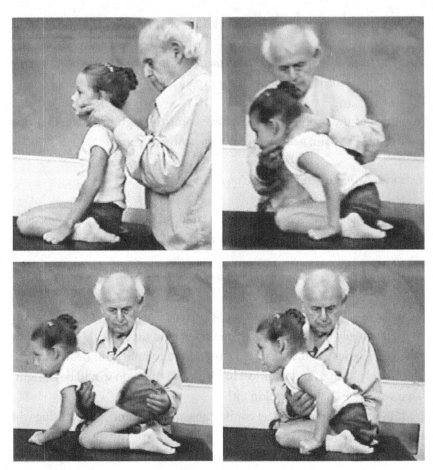

Feldenkrais working with a child, 1981.

The nervous system that works healthily makes it so that whatever you intend to do through your internal drive—or as a reaction to something happening outside of you—is performed easily, comfortably, with elegance, and doesn't take five movements in order to perform one action. My objective is to educate the person so much about himself that he doesn't find any more fault with himself. But if a person sits like this [slumping forward], and if I talk to him for ten years telling him to sit straight, he can't do it. He wouldn't know what I mean.

So how does a person become aware? You can start just by stretching out your arms and looking at their length in front of you. Which arm is longer? So, you may say, "That one's longer." Now, would you want to make it shorter? Or can you make the shorter one longer? So, if I adjust your head: now, see, the shorter one's gotten longer. So, I may say, "Look, if adjusting your head makes the shorter arm longer, maybe you actually hold your head to the other side all the time, and that's why the arm on that side is longer."

Since that is so, you will find that you move your head only to one side and that the other side is stiff in the neck and doesn't move at all. Now, how come, if you're an average healthy person? Where did you learn to move your head to one side and not to the other? And you may say, "I always had one eye better than the other." And I will say, "Oh, yeah? Is it your eyes? All right, let's close the eyes and see." And you'll find that if you move the eyes slowly to the stiff side, your stiff neck will move.

Now let's see what this man does if I tell him to get up from the chair. See, he gets up using this side because he sits on this side. He can get up only on this leg, only on this side. So, I'll say, "How would you get up on the other side? How would you do that?" Then he will find, in trying to get up on the other side, that he doesn't sit on the other hip at all. Because his head is tilted or twisted. He doesn't know that I can put this book in there under the side he doesn't sit on, but that I cannot slide the book under the hip he does sit on.

In other words, the average man in the street comes with a minor problem—like, he holds his shoulder up. When you look closer, you can see that it took a very extraordinary machine—a human brain—and circumstances of his childhood, and misunderstanding of his teachers and parents, to make that child into a being that found it was easier to be cockeyed. When he discovers that his posture is not good, he suddenly realizes the harm he has been doing to himself. His bad posture is because he has not been aware of how he has been standing, sitting, walking, holding himself. He has been cockeyed from long-standing habit.

Let's say, for example, if one side of the pelvis is raised and so the opposite shoulder is also raised so as to achieve balance—

Yes, it can't be otherwise.

Well, does it matter to you where the imbalance started, if it started in the pelvis or in the shoulder?

It never started in the pelvis or in the shoulder. It started in the brain, wherever or whatever it is.

So you are not interested in correcting this part or that part of the body?

I am not interested in correcting anybody or any part of anybody. I'll tell you something [touching the tip of his thumb to the tip of his little finger]— you'll find that this is a peculiarly human thing. No animal can do this. No ape can do this, because the ape's thumb is here on the side. Now, try to separate my fingers. If you cannot touch and hold these fingers together, you are certainly not using your full human capacity, your ability of carrying out an intention to perform. If you go into a mental hospital and find people far gone with schizophrenia, you will find few of them who can hold these fingers together. The people who can are those who have got the ability to intend and to do, which means to act normally. If I want to get up, I get up. But if somebody wants to get up and takes a half-hour, that's a nervous system which is what?

Weak.

The average person uses about ten percent of his ability.

Do you think diet is a contributory factor in the development of a person's awareness?

Certainly. If you take poison, it contributes.

Is poison different for each person?

There are some poisons that will kill anybody—a few drops of cyanide will do that. But the diet has an influence undoubtedly.

Quantity? Quality?

Both. Quantity, certainly. Quality, certainly. Try eating rotten tomatoes for a week and you will see that quality makes a difference.

There's a saying in China that at the moment of birth it is already too late to begin childhood education.

That is certainly true. Because when children come out into the world, they can already hear. In a few hours or a few days, they can already see. They can already sweat and cry. Where did they learn that? They learned it in the womb. Otherwise, how could a baby breathe coming out? He's in water. He comes out and then on the first contact with air he makes the primal cry and exhales and takes in air. Obviously he has already been having training to perform that.

In fact, we now know that children are actually taking into the lungs some amniotic liquid and regurgitating it. When they come out, the water is thrown out and the air is then taken in, and that starts respiration. The lungs have learned elasticity, everything has been formed, there is already hemoglobin, and the blood is coming through absorbing oxygen and exuding carbon dioxide.

What about artistic awareness or consciousness? How is that developed?

You know, the eunuchs were known to have made a nice choir, with strong but feminine voices. Sopranos. And their musical compositions were Vatican property and were never published. So nobody knew the music. But we know that Liszt was in the Vatican and he listened, and he went home and wrote down the music. It's said that Mozart could do the same thing.

So some few people can listen to a long, drawn-out hymn or service or composition and then go home and write it down in musical notation. But many people can't even remember a tune, or can only remember dada-da-da of the whole Ninth Symphony. But there was that extraordinary musical awareness of a Beethoven who could write when he was deaf. Of course, consciousness and awareness and being awake are three different things.

How does talent enter into this? Do you consider talent to be evidence of an inborn inclination or of a developed ability?

If you can discover talent at the age of three days and tell me that this child is going to be a general and that that child is going to be a mathematician, then I will know what talent means. We talk about talent once it's there, not before. No one could have said fifty or even twenty years ago that I would be doing *Awareness Through Movement* training or giving lectures. So, is this a talent? What do we mean by a talent? Somebody is a talented musician. At what point did he become a talented musician?

I'm uncertain of the moment. Just an attraction to music must have always been there. The talented musician must have originally been drawn to music as a form of expression. He must have liked music and felt comfortable with it and that he could develop a facility for it.

When does someone discover that?

When is the talent called a talent? It seems that would be an acknowledgment coming from the outside. Someone knowledgeable sees the talent and names it.

Can you destroy it?

Probably not entirely.

Talent is a word that grown-up people have found to describe a quality once it's there and everyone knows that it's there. Therefore, talent is not an inborn thing.

Are you saying that talent comes from what a child is exposed to in the environment?

It's not an inborn thing. The only inborn thing is tissues and a brain that's capable of learning. The talent is inculcated. You cannot be a talented pianist without ten or twenty years of playing music at a piano. You can only say that to be talented at something you must be interested in it. Because if you are not interested in music, you won't have the patience or won't find the time to practice some ten hours every day as many talented pianists need to do.

Is it conceivable that someone could grow up in some backward country without any musical instrument and at the age of sixteen go out and look for a piano? Or do you think for a person to become a musician there has to be already a piano in the home when he's growing up?

If somebody hadn't learned Chinese before the age of sixteen, he wouldn't ever learn it unless he were living in China or needed to know the language. It's the same thing with the piano. If an Eskimo was born in an igloo and never heard of or saw a piano in his life, and then you brought him at the age of sixteen to the Juilliard, you would see that no teacher there would undertake to teach him. The teacher would think it's a waste of time. And why should the Eskimo play the piano?

But if the child were seven years old would it be different?

No. For an Eskimo to be brought to the Juilliard at the age of seven, it's too late. An Eskimo child being brought to the Juilliard and seeing these people fiddling, and those others playing brass, and others drumming, he would just be driven crazy. He would find himself running away, saying, "They're a band of mad people."

Yet he could be very musical. He could detect the movement of a white bear on the ice that all of Juilliard would never detect. He wouldn't be called a talented musician, yet if he'd been born here he could have been a musician. And by the way, if you think about this a little bit, does a talented musician also not have to have somewhere in his guts a desire for the public to hear him? And why does a talented musician want a public? Why can't he learn to play the piano and go to the seashore and play for himself?

He desires the performance. He wants that public contact.

A talented pianist must have an audience that can understand that talented pianist. Otherwise, he wouldn't be able to sustain the capacity to practice for ten years. For what? And who would build pianos if there were not a public interested in hearing the piano? When somebody can play so that the public is interested, he then has the potential to develop into a genius— and be given a lot of money, and so on. A pianist needs that.

And he needs an audience.

In an Eskimo child there is no sense of that need for an understanding public. He would not comprehend what you wanted for him with the piano, why he should torture himself ten hours a day—unless you introduce him to the public, and educate him, and make him into a Western child. At seven years, it's too late. You will have to bring in a lot of psychiatrists, and they would not know what to do with the child.

What do you think of the Hindu concept of karma, of a former life having some influence on what a person becomes in this life?

I don't believe it. I don't deal with things I don't know. I don't go into things that are impossible to know, that I have no means of knowing. I know about as much as you do about things that are impossible to know. I also know as much as people who claim that they know, but they don't know either.

What about the effects of heredity?

Heredity can be quite well defined. Heredity means that if you were born in Japan to natives of that country, then your eyes are Japanese.

You don't mean that heredity is just physiological?

Not only physiological. The tissues of the brain are also involved. There is the quality of the brain: the way it can learn, how much it can learn, what sort of retention it has. That's all heredity.

What role do parents play in who the child becomes?

What can I say? If we didn't have parents, we would be all right. But if you think about it, most parents are actually much better than not. They have two or three cuckoo things that they do to their children, things they do wrongly. And generally they don't do them wrongly intentionally. They themselves are probably a bit cuckoo, having been wronged by somebody else before.

How many wrong things can a mother do to a child? Or tell a child? "Be careful," or "Don't do that, you silly," or something. She can have fifteen faults in her behavior. But do you know what it takes to bring a person to the age of twenty? How many sleepless nights did she have with that baby having its thumb there, its teeth, diarrhea, and childhood diseases? And she managed to get it to school and clothe it. Even if you get bad parents, the badness is one percent of what they do good. But that one percent can be just like putting a spoonful of sand in a Rolls-Royce. The spoonful of sand can spoil the Rolls-Royce. That's parents.

10

The Extraordinary Story of How Moshe Feldenkrais Came to Study Judo

Interview with Dennis Leri

This interview took place during the San Francisco Teacher Training Program in 1977 in a group setting. The atmosphere was informal and conversational. Dennis Leri, who led the interview, was one of Moshe Feldenkrais's original American students and has become one of the most respected Feldenkrais teachers of his generation. He is a longtime practitioner of the martial arts; his background includes aikido, northern-style kung fu, and Chen-style T'ai Chi. Dennis was accompanied in the interview by Mia Segal, Robert Volberg, Frank Wildman, Anna Johnson, and Jerry Karzen (all involved with the ongoing teacher training) and Charles Alston, a Yang-style T'ai Chi instructor. The piece appeared originally in *The Feldenkais Journal* in 1986.—*Ed.*

D. LERI ET AL.: *What has your history been in the martial arts?*

MOSHE: Oh, I could write a book of it. It's an extraordinary story. . . . If you want it in short, it's like this: You know that I went to Israel when I was very young; then it wasn't Israel, it was Palestine. There was a British mandate, and the British being very great experts in politics use that rule that the Romans invented: divide and conquer. It means that if you want to occupy a place without having to keep a million soldiers there, all you [the British] have to do is say to Mr. X that Mr. Y said to you whatever, or you say one thing to Mr. X, and something else to Mr. Y, and then in five weeks the two bite each other and they continue that forever. And all you have to say is that you [Mr. X] are right. No, you [Mr. Y] are right, no, you [Mr. X] are right … [Laughter] … and for twenty-five years you can rule with no expense, but with a lot of bloodshed. Whose blood? The people who kill each other. They did the same thing in India. They do that the world over. And all the other people, if you think only the English do it, all those who rule other people do that. There is no other way of doing it. That's the experience of the world. Now, the British mandate in Israel was like that. And trouble between Jews and Arabs continues until today with the fomented hatred that the British introduced between the Jews and the Arabs. Because Arabs and Jews throughout their history lived like cousins together. And during the Golden Era of our culture, the Maimonides Era, lived our greatest poets and the Arabs' greatest poets and mathematicians; Maimonides wrote some of his books in Arabic and some in Hebrew. And so did the Arabs. They knew Hebrew. It was the Golden Age for both of them. And they never had any quarrel. And then came the British, and they produced a hatred which for two thousand years wasn't there, between Jews and Arabs. And so when I arrived in Palestine, we were a small group of people. …

If I keep telling you the story like this, it will only take us two days. So what happens later is that the British would begin some kind of trouble and while Jews and Arabs were hitting each other, the British never intervened. They would send the police force to make peace, but the police force was more concerned with their horses than with the blood that was shed. They would come to the outskirts of the city, and they would stop there for two hours to feed their horses. They would come into the city when there were already fifty dead on either side. Then they would come and disarm those who were there with weapons. …

Now, there were many young people like myself; I was then sixteen years old. I was like everybody else. We decided we will die, but these [damn] British won't be here, and we won't be pitted against the Arabs as enemies forever. And so we all formed the Haganah,* which means the self-defense

---

*The Haganah began as informal, locally organized defense units to guard Jewish farms and kibbutzim in Palestine. It started in 1920 and originally was poorly armed with little central organization. As time passed the group became more organized, with a much larger membership. Here Feldenkrais is referring to the early period of the Haganah in the 1920s.

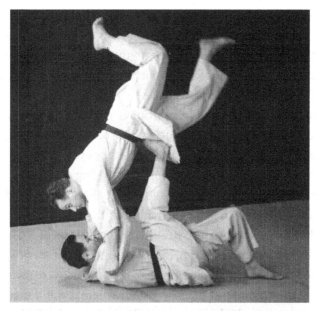

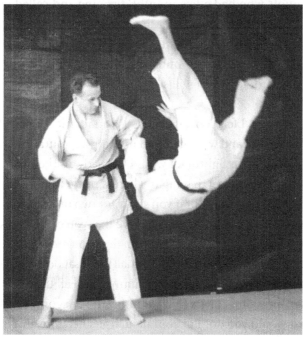

Feldenkrais being thrown by M. Kawaishi (top).
Feldenkrais executing a judo throw (bottom).

force. We were three hundred young men and we had nothing—we didn't even have knives, but only sticks. So, we put ourselves together, we started learning how to use our hands, sticks, anything that comes to your hand, so as to be able to take care of the population who couldn't defend themselves at all.

And we had some boy who came from Germany who was an expert in jujitsu and he gave us the first lessons in jujitsu. After some time, we were all big experts in jujitsu. We were training every evening. But then it was quiet for a few months, so people stopped training and gave it up. Then when trouble started again, it turned out that all those who didn't know jujitsu, who hadn't trained in that way, none of them were injured or killed because they ran away and hid. But the big experts went against knives and swords with naked hands or with a stick, and half of them were killed, or wounded. Look! The people who were not trained were saved because they ran, or they didn't put their necks out where it was dangerous. But these silly idiots who had a few months' training and called themselves experts because in the gymnasium using mattresses, they could do something to somebody who was half attacking and half not, half of them were killed. It's just like if you do a month of aikido and you try to fight somebody with a sword, then you will see what your aikido is worth. So, that was that.

I couldn't take it. I felt, look, this jujitsu is an idiotic system. Obviously, if I trained all my life and was interested in being a samurai and focused all my life on training, on fighting, I would be ready all the time. And even when walking in the street, having my hands ready to draw my sword, I would know I am immune. But if you study for two months and then have two years without training and then believe that you can take a sword out of someone's hands who wants to kill you, then you are an innocent idiot. And your chances of success are [damn small]. So I sat down and said, look, I am going to propose something very funny. From all the tricks of jujitsu I learned, say, most of them are worth nothing. If I am going to hit you with a knife, what would you do? Put your hand up? Therefore, this is the point to begin. Now, I will train you with that movement only, until you, not thinking or not knowing anything, you will still protect your head and your throat and your own body against any attack, building off the first movement that you do spontaneously.

And then I went and took a group of people, and I took a knife and I attacked each of them and I photographed them. And I retained their first move, and I found that for certain, if you really attack, nobody stands there and gets the knife. He does something to protect himself. He doesn't attack you, but he substitutes an arm for the head, the throat, the back. If you try to hit somebody, you will see what they do; they won't stand with arms down, facing you, defenseless. When you hit them with a stick, they will turn their backs toward you and protect their heads and let you hit them on the back. And therefore, most people, even in the movies, when they show people hit with sticks for punishment, you will see they will always let you hit them on the back. And the back, it's painful. But it is not dangerous, unless, of course, you break every bone, which is possible. But even if you break his every bone, he won't die; he will die later, but not on the spot. So that was the idea, to find out what was the first movement one does. And I built a system of defense for any sort of attack where the first movement is not what you think to do, what you decide to do, but what you actually do when you are frightened. And I said, all right, let's see now, we will train the people so that [the] end of their first spontaneous movement is where we must start. And let us see now, we'll train them [for] three months like we did before, give them a year off without training regularly, and then a year afterwards, try to attack again. And of course, the year afterwards, the first defensive movement they did, once they did their spontaneous first movement, was the continuation of the first movement. It was a remarkable thing. Most of the people knew what to do immediately without previous notice. They did it, and I was as pleased as punch and, of course, I got another few guys in the Haganah to help me and we worked about two or three years and perfected that idea. I submitted the thing to the direction of the Haganah, which at that time was a secret group; nobody knew their names lest they [be] exposed to the British and be hanged. And I remember until today, they gave me 25 pounds sterling, which was in 1921 equivalent today to $100,000. And with those 25 pounds, I published a book in Hebrew which contained that system and which was distributed to every man in the

Haganah so those not in Tel Aviv but in other colonies everywhere could learn with the book what to do. There were pictures, everything.

The British, if the book fell into their hands and they knew that I wrote it, they would probably arrest me and ask me who the leaders of the Haganah were and so on. So the day the book was published, I was in France. And there was a man who was Colonel Keech, a British colonel, who actually gave us the 25 pounds to do it. So that was done. I left. I went to France to study mechanical and electrical engineering, and I completely forgot about that damned thing because I was preoccupied with my studies.

Now, one day, the people in the hotel where I lived knew that I knew some tricks as you saw here [Moshe had demonstrated some of the techniques he developed.—DL.] The caretaker of the hotel knew that I was from Palestine, it wasn't Israel yet, and that I knew something about self-defense and that I could throw people, immobilize them, do things to them. And one day he brought to me a newspaper entirely dedicated to sports. He showed me, look, it says there's to be a demonstration where a Japanese minister of education, Professor Kano,* is going to demonstrate judo in Paris. The Japanese ambassador to France would be present also. I didn't know who Kano was, but I was really impressed that a man who does some judo, which I didn't know about, but which I understood to be a martial art connected with Jujitsu or something, is doing a demonstration, so I wanted to see.... Actually, at the beginning I said I would have to prepare for exams and I don't want to be bothered. Then the people said, "Why don't you go? Surely it may be something interesting." So I decided to go and have a look. Because of the minister of education and the Japanese ambassador ... there was a security guard there and every person who went in had to have an invitation and they checked for it. Now, I had nothing, so when I went there I couldn't get in.

When I arrived there and found nothing doing, I couldn't go in, I was insulted, peeved. After all, I am interested in such affairs, I was going there

---

*Jigoro Kano (1860–1938) was the renowned and highly respected founder and creator of judo. He is often referred to as Professor Kano as he worked for much of his life as an educator.

not because the ambassador is there, but because I want to see what sort of thing judo is. I had not the faintest idea. But it certainly concerned martial arts and therefore I was interested. So I returned home and took my Hebrew book with the pictures, about this self-defense business, and went back to the door. I had a card, and I put on the card "You see that I am interested in and studied jujitsu, and I am interested in seeing what and how judo is done. Would you see to it that I can see the demonstration?" and I wrote it to Professor Kano. I told the officer to go on and give it to him. I didn't have much hope that he would see it, and I didn't know if he could read French. He could read Japanese; maybe he doesn't know what it is, French, but I hoped for the best. And I stood there and waited about a quarter of an hour and then had the surprise of my life. A Japanese gentleman came out and opened the door for me, pulled the people apart, and brought me into the hall and gave me quite a respectable seat—not tops, but a place where I could see everything. [Laughter]

So I sat there and watched. I watched, I couldn't . . . it looked very funny to me. Funny was this: Kano was a tiny little man and was old and his face had wrinkles and all that, and I saw behind him the Japanese ambassador, Sugimura, who was about six-foot-five, something extraordinary for a Japanese, bigger than you and larger, a tremendous figure. And this little Kano, if Kano stood up to say something, the Japanese ambassador stood up and he wouldn't sit until this chap Kano sits down. So I said to myself, very funny. Because somebody can do some tricks in jujitsu or something, why should the ambassador look at him like he was godlike. Actually, it seemed ridiculous, I couldn't understand. The French minister sat there and he also couldn't understand what's happening.

Then, two chaps were brought in and one of them was Kotani* and the other one, Ida. She [pointing to Mia] was in Japan; she was there when I met Kotani and told him, "You're Kotani and you did the demonstration in 1932 in Paris." He just couldn't understand who knew that he was in Paris

---

*Sumiyuki Kotani (1903–1991) was one of Professor Kano's original students and often accompanied him for international demonstrations. He was one of the few people to be given the rank of tenth dan by Kano.

in 1932* giving a demonstration. But to me the demonstration was an extraordinary thing. That's why it sticks in my memory and why I knew him. Ida is one of the greatest in ground work, ground wrestling, in judo. In Japan, there are two books by Ida, which are a rarity even in Japan—wonderful books. And although he was a small little chap he could do extraordinary things. Now these two chaps were there because Kotani studied mathematics in Cambridge. What Ida did, I didn't know, but they said actually Kano invited those two because they were high-grade judo men and between them they gave a demonstration. They seemed silly idiots; one and then the other would fall, would fly through the air and did what looked like no work at all. And obviously it was prearranged business, because they really didn't do anything and then a chap would fly and then they would make noises, shout "Ha!" and make a throw. It looked completely cockeyed. . . . I believed actually that it was prearranged, that it was a kata, a practiced form, and not a randori or freestyle match. I didn't believe in it, but the two were supposedly some of the best. One was sixth dan in the Kodokan** and one was fifth dan, and they were both champions of Japan, twice before that. They were both extraordinary fellows. And their work in fact looked like playing. The platform on which they were doing it was like a ring; they were in the whole ring; they were everywhere. It was a magnificent sight; to this day I can always remember how I didn't know what I was seeing. So I looked and then the old little man came out, came into the ring, and started doing judo with the two of them. He tried to do randori with each one of them. These were two strong guys with terrible, fierce muscles and wonderful movement, and then there is an old man of about sixty-five or seventy, but I couldn't tell what his age was. You know an old Japanese, how could you tell? And he does something very funny; he takes that young, strong guy and makes a simple move, and holds him there and says, "@!!*#" . . . and throws him. Surely the other chap must let him do it, and then he

---

* Feldenkrais may be misremembering here as other sources put Kano and Feldenkrais meeting in September 1933.–*Ed.*

   **Dan refers to black belt level, so sixth dan means sixth degree black belt. The Kodokan is the headquarters of the judo world.

threw him again. I believed that that was real eyewash, and I thought to myself, Kano, you are such a big expert, you would live ten seconds in my hands. [Laughter] And I really believed it, because you know I had real experience in battle with shooting and throwing knives and stones. And this looked to me to be a phony theatrical business. Therefore, obviously, I could lick them.

Now, I had nothing particular to do, so while the demonstration was going on, I sat there and watched. When it was over, everybody went away. The audience was there by invitation of the minister and everybody was in tuxedos and beautiful, and I was like an ordinary citizen. I didn't want to push myself among them; I said, well, all right, I'm in no hurry; after they go out, I will go comfortably out, which I did. I intended to go home. I was rather disappointed. It was nice to see, but I didn't think that there was anything to learn from this show. So, I began to go out, and then suddenly somebody came to me and said, "Excuse me, are you Feldenkrais?" I said yes. "Professor Kano asked whether you would be willing to have dinner with him." I nearly fell off my seat. I couldn't believe it, and I thought it was a joke. Have dinner? So I said, yes, but my wife was at home and I told her that the demonstration wouldn't last later than ten o'clock or something like that. I'll be back as soon as it's over, I'd said. [To Jerry Karzen] Well, I had very much nicer food there. [Jerry brought some blintzes to Moshe to eat and told him they were getting cold. Moshe obviously enjoyed the memory of that meal in Paris more than the prospect of some cold deli blintzes.] [Laughter] Anyway, they said, "Will you please wait here." And a big Rolls-Royce comes up while people are still leaving and Kano gets in first and the Japanese ambassador stands there and helps me to get in and there I sit between Kano and this Japanese ambassador. I felt like sitting on charcoal. I didn't know what to say, didn't know what to do.

You must not forget that I was a young man, coming from a small, provincial place into Paris, finding myself suddenly at the summit of what I could've never imagined. I really didn't know what to do. Though I tried to be as composed as I could, I assure you I was covered with cold sweat and warm sweat several times during that ride.

How did you communicate?

He speaks French and English. Where did they take us? In Paris, there is a big hotel where all Japanese visitors of good standing go. It is a very expensive, exclusive hotel. Now, we arrived there, the Japanese ambassador got out, and opened the door for me, and showed me out. We went into the hotel, and he asked me, "What would you like for dinner?" "I don't know what I ..." I said. "Anything you have." He said, "You know, I like trout: I would like a trout for dinner." At that time, for me, it wasn't much of a dinner to eat a trout. I was a very strong man and young. I could eat five trout just to begin with as an appetizer. Well, I had to do what they did. We went into a very big hall about the size of a basketball court, and it was covered with tatami mats like in a normal dojo. There was a small table on the floor, funny sort of way of sitting to eat I thought, but I sat on the floor too. And Kano sat in front of me and the two huge guys, extraordinary fellows, one with a mustache, you could see he had tremendous power, served us. I remember it until today. You see, suppose you sit here, that's me, and Kano sits over there, and the big one comes to put something on the table and asks to pass making hand gestures. I couldn't figure out what he wanted, so I made with the hand too. [Laughter] I didn't know what he wanted, so he made with the hand again and then bent like that, he bowed. He made the hand pass between me and the table. Then every time he brought something to the table, he did exactly the same thing, pom pom pom. All right, everything new and queer, so, and there I sat with Kano and I didn't know what he wanted. I couldn't understand why all this wining and dining.

And then he told me stories of his students like ... Nagaoka.* At that time, Nagaoka meant to me exactly like if you told me Gerald Ford. [Laughter] So, keeping things rolling, I said, "Who's Nagaoka?" He said, "He is the chief instructor of the Kodokan." Then, around 1930, there were two judo greats, Nagaoka and Mifune.** Nagaoka was the most powerful man

---

*Hidekazu Nagaoka (1876–1952) was a legendary judoka and head of the Kodokan for many years. He was one of the few men to achieve tenth dan.

**Kyuzo Mifune (1883–1965) is considered by many to be the best judo technician after Kano. He was one of the few judoka to receive the rank of tenth dan.

in the Kodokan and Mifune, the fastest, the best in quality. Kind of a small chap, but he could beat anybody. Actually I heard very many very long stories; Kano told me extraordinary things. He told me about Mifune afterwards, later; we met about twelve times afterwards. So, he told me that Mifune was a born fighter and that two or three times every year, he had to go to the police and take him out of prison. Wherever there was a brawl, wherever there was fighting, Mifune was there and usually an ambulance had to take away a dozen people and the police would arrest him. [Laughter] You see? Then Kano as the Undersecretary of State for Education in Japan had to use his influence. He told me that he had to get Mifune out of prison perhaps thirty times in his life.

But here they appeared as two nice gentlemen, but they were dressed in a funny sort of way, with black belts and judo *gis* [white practice outfits— *Ed.*], which I saw for the first time in my life. Both of them had on Japanese sandals. They served dinner for both of us. At the table were Kano and myself. Then after we had eaten they asked me who I was and what I was doing in Paris. I was astonished to find that he knew what a Bible is. I told him that I was from Palestine. He knew that there was a Bible, that there were Jews in the world. I thought the Japanese wouldn't know a thing about it, but obviously he was a cultured man and who knew a lot of things. He asked how and why I went to Israel, who my parents were. I told him all my life history, but I had no idea what he wanted from me.

Then when the dinner was finished, he took my Hebrew book and said to me, "I can understand this even if I can't read it." He said, "But here is something I can't understand. Show me how do you do that technique" [a knife-disarming technique]. It was one of the parts of my book, my own invention, a modified jujitsu trick. And that was in the book. So he obviously had looked at the pictures. He said, "This is very funny, I know eleven *ryūs*—means eleven different schools of martial arts—in Japan that I learned before I started judo. I learned eleven *ryūs*, and I know all the tricks that exist, and I've never seen that trick. Where did you get it?" So I told him the story I told you of how I did it. He looked bewildered and said, "That's wonderful. Show me again." So I did it with a real knife that was on the table, and of course, threw the knife away. I was strong and quick and I threw the knife. It flew away, half a mile. And then he clapped loudly and Nagaoka came and Kano gave him the knife and said, "You try it with him; I want to see it again." And I did the same thing again. And he saw it and approved. He didn't make any overt display ... you know, Japanese are impassive. But, he obviously was interested.

Then he read on in the book and said, "This is very interesting, but look, what you show here [a choke-hold], it is no good." I said, "What do you mean it's no good? Why is it no good?" I said, in my experience, I had never had anyone who was capable of getting out of that except by being dead. He said, "Hmm, no good." I said, "No good? Well, you show me why it's not good." The technique was that I get you on the floor, and use my hands against your throat and with the help of a jacket or anything like that plus putting full power into it, you have a minute to live. A minute, a second. You see black immediately. You choke. He said, "Try it on me." And as I was more powerful than this little man, I thought, with an old man like that I must be gentle. So I did it slowly, and then I found that he just didn't mind what I was doing and so pushed as hard as I could, and believe it or not, I blacked out. I didn't realize actually what was happening. He said, "You see, it's no good." [ha ha] So I asked him what happened; I didn't know; I saw black. So he explained to me, "Look, strangulation," he talks in French. "Strangulation, pardon? Comme ça? Pardon, comme ça? You cannot strangle anybody by straightening your arm." I said, "But I always do it and it always works." He said, "Yeah, but ordinary people don't know how to defend themselves. Try it again." And I wasn't really keen on trying again, because I never had anything like that happen to me before until then. I said, "All right, I'll try again." And while I did, I saw that he had his hands completely free, and that he used my strength to strangle me. Not just choke me, cut off my air, but cut the flow of blood to the brain. It felt terrible because something on which I relied, my power and the way I did the technique, suddenly I found the more I pushed, the more I strangled myself. I blacked out. Not he. And I didn't notice just because it was so perfectly done; I didn't even realize that he held me. I saw him holding his hands, putting his fingers there, but what do I care? I have him in a grip which I was sure will finish him off. And he said, "You are an intelligent man. I must check this knife technique out. But you can see your book is not very good. But it is very interesting." It was two o'clock when we finished.

I arrived home at 3 a.m., and my wife was very worried. She had gone to the place of the demonstration, but everything was closed and I wasn't there. I wanted to phone, but what can you do? I didn't dare. I didn't think I could ask to phone. I wanted to phone. I thought of it twenty times, but somehow I felt it was a hassle. I would have to pay him for the phone call. And it's minor things like that that make life difficult. So, I sat there and I wanted to go home and I had to go to school. I was studying engineering· then. I had to go to school early in the morning, and I hadn't prepared for my math examination, as I told you. I listened and was interested, but wanted to go home. At the end, Kano explained to me why you have to strangle like that, the principle of it. And he told me that he will take my knife-disarming trick, and try it out for a year in the Kodokan to determine why it wasn't used. He thought maybe it was too dangerous, or maybe that it won't work, or that it's easy to defend against. But he was intrigued that he had never seen it. It was late at night, half past two. He wanted to go to bed, so he wanted to send me away. And I said, "Can I get a taxi, because there is no underground, and I need to get home?" "Oh," he said, and the ambassador's Rolls-Royce with the driver came around and took me home. I sat there alone in that auto and decided that it was fun. My wife was still sitting up when I arrived home. She was worried. She hadn't known what to do. So it took me another few hours to tell her the whole story and I had a sleepless night that night.

I forgot about it. It was a nice experience and that's that. Two days later, there's a phone call from the Japanese Embassy telling me that Kano left a letter for me and that the Japanese ambassador would like to see me. I thought, Oh, I haven't got time to waste one evening after the other with such business. I saw what I saw and let's be finished with it. But I couldn't dare not to answer, So I phoned. He talked very friendly to me, as if we knew each other ever since, and told me, "Look, Professor Kano has left for London, but will be back tomorrow and he asked me to invite you for lunch because he wants to talk to you. I will be there too." Now this time, I didn't know what to do. I couldn't go to lunch dressed in my usual stuff. So, I went and bought a kind of tuxedo with a tie, which I never wore again. I didn't like it. Dressed like that I was as clumsy as an ape. I thought I must be posh to go to lunch with them. These chaps talked to me as if I were a real guest. They were very polite, they let me sit first and so on. I thought, "What sort of trouble have I gotten myself into?" And then Kano tells me, "Look, I think you're the kind of man who will succeed in bringing judo to Europe. We have tried three or four times and it was a failure. We have sent Ida, the man you saw in the demonstration. He started with a big group, and in six months he had nobody, he had to close. We had several other experts try also and it didn't work. I believe that you have the stuff, but you can't go on teaching that junk you have in your book. You have to learn proper judo."

I said, "I have no time to learn anything properly because I am doing my university studies." He said, "We will see to it so that you have the time you need. We will send you to an expert from Japan who'll teach you judo. And I will see to it that you are formed into a good judo man. And with his help, after you have been graded, you will start a club. And I will send you four rolls of film where you will see judo done by me, by Nagaoka, by Yokoyama* and Mifune, and that's the best judo that has ever been filmed. We will test that trick of yours. If it is really good, you will be the first white man ever to have a judo trick on the curriculum of the Kodokan. And meanwhile the Japanese ambassador will see to your needs while you're learning judo; whatever you need, phone him. He will do everything you wish to help your progress." That was how I got into judo. And on those cinemas there are some very nice things, and there is something very funny there, too. The black belt, first dan, fights the second dan and then you see that the first dan has not a blooming chance. You can see that; the second dan does what he wants. And you see this big hero doing everything, then he gets with a third dan and suddenly he is played with. Because at that time, the dans took five to seven years to get and people were really formed, not like now—you get the belt after paying so much and being six months in the dojo. To get the sixth dan, you had to be one in five million people, the best. Now, anybody

---

*Yokoyama Sakujiro (1864–1914) was one of Professor Kano's earliest students and head of the Kodokan for many years.

who goes to a club, in a year or a year and a half, they get to be a black belt. It doesn't mean much anymore. A black belt today is a second-rate achievement. You can see even the higher grades in the Olympic Games. It's the ugliest sight I've ever seen, worse than boxing, worse than wrestling. Both of them are nicer than the judo performed in the Olympic Games. Kano, if he saw that, he would die.

Why has the quality of judo gone down?

Because so long as Kano was alive, he didn't allow judo into the Olympic Games, and he didn't allow weight distinctions. Skill is the final thing. In the Olympic Games you have weight categories. Because, there, like in wrestling, they believe that a lightweight cannot beat a heavyweight. Now they have that weight system which requires a small man to fight a small man, never a big one. So you see those fellows using strength to push each other, and they don't do any judo; they do a parody of judo. It's against the grain of judo. It's ugly to see and inefficient. And Kano said, "So long as I am alive, judo won't have weight distinctions and if the day comes that it becomes a part of the Olympic Games, it will become a wash-out. Judo is finished with inclusion into the Olympic Games." And, unfortunately, he was right.

Is the entire body of judo teaching very different now than it was?

Completely, even in Japan. Because, you see, the Japanese are very proud of their judo. But now it's all a question of violent power, which is against the grain of judo. Judo is a school where you use your opponent's strength; and therefore, it's based on moving, not on resisting, not on pushing back against a push. Who's going to push someone stronger and get somewhere? Kano was a tiny little man who could throw any wrestler who pushed him, anytime, immediately. And that's the principle, that if someone pushed him, he would sink under him, and the chap who would fall over Kano's body only because he's pushing. Kano would come under his hips and help his push. He disappears from under the push so smoothly that the other person

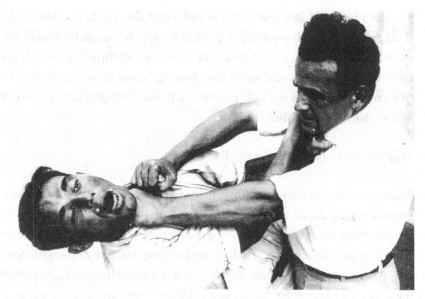

Feldenkrais choking an unknown opponent.

goes over without knowing how or why. Nowadays, they push back, and nobody is nimble enough with that *tai sabaki*, you call it in judo—it means the mobility of the hips, turning the back to the front—nobody is nimble enough to do that. They are not trained anymore like that.

The real champions, they never fought. They came there to beat you, not to fight you. They were there to show you that you are no match for them and that was the idea. They didn't go in for fighting. One of them would go there to show you that you were nothing, that his skill is so much greater than yours that you have not a chance in a million. In fact, he will let you do whatever kind of hold on him, just to show you he can get out of it. My teacher would lie on the floor and leave his throat exposed and a stick would be put to his throat with two people holding the stick down, pressing the stick onto his throat. Anybody would be dead in a second. He would lie there, and before you knew it, he was out from under the stick, out of their hold. He could do that ten times running and you still couldn't stop him from doing it. And the thing is extremely simple, but you have to have the skill, the stamina to do it. He would do it to the right and the left, anytime

142

he wanted. It looks like a godlike ability, but then he teaches you how to do it. Now any judo man today if you put a stick to his throat, he will die. [Chuckle]

Are there still people who do teach it in that old style?

Oh, yes, there are some old men in Japan who are just as peeved about this as myself. They look at these young, silly idiots who are spoiling their judo heritage, which was unique in the world, and who make out of it shit. There are many people who ...

Are they only in Japan?

Well, there are some of my students, like Glen in Paris: he's a very small man and he's sixth dan today. He was trained by me and by Kawaishi* and he is small. He could beat people three times his weight. And even today, although he is merely a few years younger than I, he still can beat the best teacher in Paris. There are several others like that, but not many. They are dying.

You were talking the other day about the ki, chi, that kind of thing. I'd like to know what you think about that.

Ki and chi are the same thing. You better, about ki and chi, ask Chinese people or other Asian people. Because they talk about ki and chi. I can tell

---

*Mikinosuke Kawaishi (1899–1969) moved to Paris in 1936 and began teaching at the judo school Feldenkrais had opened in the Latin Quarter of Paris. Kawaishi was a fourth dan at this time and already an experienced instructor. He and Feldenkrais had a fruitful collaboration including running the school together, founding the French Judo association, and shooting many action photographs that were later used in both Feldenkrais's and Kawaishi's books. In some accounts Feldenkrais is written out of the history of European judo and all credit given to Kawaishi, despite the fact that Feldenkrais was responsible for opening the first school there in 1933. This has been remedied in a recent definitive history written by Michel Brousse, *Le judo: son histoire, ses succès.*

you only that Koizumi,* when he wanted to talk about it, there was an international congress of judo black belts in London and I was one of them. There were about five hundred there. And we had a special course conducted by Koizumi. And then in the middle of the course, on the fifth day, suddenly he says, "Now I am going to talk to you about the most important principle in judo training, about the *saika tanden:* Some people call it *tan tien,* the seat of chi, ki, or whatever you like, but it's the *saika tanden* in Japanese. But Feldenkrais, come here," and he said to the whole assemblage, "I believe he will talk to you about the *saika tanden* more sensibly and in a way in which you'll understand. It is something which I feel and know, but which I cannot explain." And then he let me explain that for the people there. And he wrote the preface to my book. The thing is this, when you talk of such matters in my way, nobody will take it for ki and chi or anything you like. You see, most people talk about that as if it's a mysterious kind of thing in the lower abdomen with all sorts of metaphysical meanings and powers. I have no connection with that. And therefore, my way of thinking is actually a useless thing to such people. If you challenge them on that they say, "Ah, what does he know? He is only a scientist."

But this is only a semantic difference, isn't it?

Oh, no. A semantic difference? No. Ghosts are a semantic difference? Ghosts are something which if you believe in and you are afraid of a ghost, you will never go into a haunted house.

Yes, but you must know.... It's not semantic, but you must know from your practice something, the importance of this, what they call in the language, tanden.

Of course, I know.

---

*Gunji Koizumi (1885–1965) was the first high-ranking judoka to settle and teach in Europe. He founded the British Judo Association and taught all over Europe. He was Feldenkrais's judo instructor and they had a close relationship. Koizumi wrote the introduction to Feldenkrais's book *Higher Judo.*

And their description of it, while it may be . . .

My description of it is only in movement; I am not concerned with any of the other things.

But does it not come to the same thing?

No, it doesn't, because, you see, in the one, if you say you've got chi, many people would try to be like you and do like you, and if they fail will say, "Oh, I could never get chi." To get chi, you have to possess moral courage; you have to be connected with the higher spheres of things. Therefore, you find that this is an impediment in the learning. [To a questioner] Have you chi?

I could not say that.

Oh, therefore, if you can't say it, that's what I'm talking about. You can work twenty years and you don't show it. You're not sure if you have it or you don't. Because if it's a mysterious quantity, then you must deserve it, you must be a part of an elite group, or you must be born in China. How will you get chi if it's a metaphysical thing that nobody knows what it is? Well, it's a quality like psychic healing: if you're a healer, you're a healer. If you don't heal, you are not. Now, chi is the same thing. Either you've got it or you ain't got it. If you've got *it*, you've got it. If you ain't got it, you ain't got it. [Laughter] It's almost like *est.*

But what you're talking about is different.

Yes. I told you. In movement, I can show you what chi is, what ki is, on you or anybody else. Can you see that my notions on breathing are different from anything you heard before and you will ever hear? You can see it, you can test it, on yourself, and there is a marked difference between the one and the other, provided that you can make the contrast.

Okay, for example, in martial arts training, in aikido, where they have the notion of the unbendable arm or they talk about focusing somewhere, like a couple of inches below the navel and a couple inches inside the lower abdomen, and then having your weight underside and not being stiff, but not relaxed, but having your attention ...

Well, I don't know that it's a few inches here and a few inches there. It has to do with the full organization of your body; you can see it in whatever you do. You actually get chi through using the pelvis and the lower abdominal muscles, the strong muscles of the body, as a unit concentrated from where all push or pull is issued. The rest of the body and the arms needn't be powerful. It is not a muscle; it is not a point. It has nothing to do with this point, because if it were a point ... Look, if you move your body like that, the point is gone [makes a move to demonstrate, a shift in the center of gravity to outside the body]. A point a few inches there, a few inches here, if you go there, you will find that it is full of shit, literally. [Laughter] That point is full of shit. And this is the point of chi.

So, will you teach us this organization?

What do you want it for? You don't want to fight. What do you want?

Is it used only in fighting or is it a whole organization that is serving you in any other action?

Of course, it serves me. I believe a dancer is not a dancer without that reorganization. That is why most dancers are half-cooked dancers.

Why would we go through life without it?

You wouldn't know it. And nobody would do the amount of work that is necessary to get it because they will have to change their dancing.

But people like us can learn it?

I am teaching you whether you want it or not. The improvement in your movement that you get moving the head free so that the pelvis can produce the necessary power, that's all. What did Kano do? That's all. He stands there, you can't push him. If he wants to push you, you go wherever he wants. So the mysterious development of chi is efficient use of the equipment that everybody has. It is that question which needs, in order to understand it, a tremendous amount of knowledge. And as usual, it's easier to teach people without teaching understanding, by saying, look, this is it, imitate me. Look, I stand here unmovable. You can't move me. Now push me, you can't push me. If I push you, you move.

Now and then they have you send the chi down to the ground and bring it back up, each way. It is a marvelous technique. But you know in a way, it's interesting that they teach that way because, if the motor cortex is responsible for directing the organization of the body, then to tell someone to send their energy down would cause them to organize their body differently and so their weight would be more difficult to move. But, if you say you send your energy . . . how do you send energy here or there? Show me any instance where you can send energy anywhere. In our work we can do something with awareness and without awareness, something just purely done in a mechanical fashion and we can also pay attention to making some movement. So I see the concept of ki and chi as an incredible impediment to learning and I see people in classes, aikido and kung fu and whatever, and it's just a struggle. They can never get it. They never get it because the idea of chi or ki is preposterous. How can you get it if it's a point in your stomach? What would you do with such a point? What can you do with it? What change will it make to you? Now, it sounds [like] a mysterious kind of super power that you get from somewhere in the point in your stomach, and that point, described properly, is the duodenum lying there and is literally full of shit.

Your teacher, and Kano, were trained with that notion in a cultural matrix that allowed them to not view it all so mysteriously.

Oh, certainly. And Kano, when he had already a school where most of [the] people could beat anybody in Japan, he brought a boy that was fourteen years old into the dojo and none of those big experts could throw him

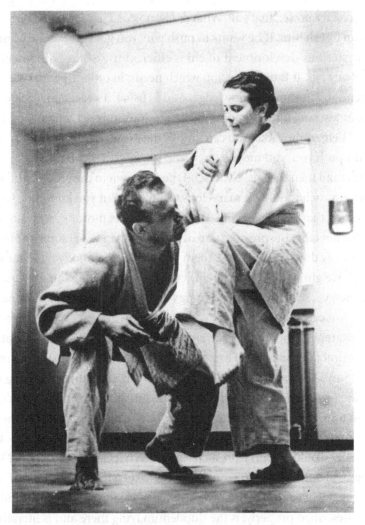

Feldenkrais being thrown by his sister, Malka Silice.

because that boy had a natural what they called *tai sabaki,* meaning hips moving away. You could never break his balance; he always slid away, whatever you did to him, like a cat. Balance. He was always coming back on his feet, whatever you did to him. And most people couldn't get a grip on him; if you pulled him he was with you, but you could never make his pelvis go outside the feet, whatever you did, and they were very peeved. They said, look, judo is no good. He said, "You are no good." This chap will be here until you learn to do like he does, or learn how to fight, that sort of thing. Only then will you have a better *saika tanden* than he. He is better than any one of you; therefore, you have to learn.

If you were to start a judo school today, would you begin with your work, Awareness Through Movement?

Well, I can tell you that I have been teaching judo exactly in the same way. The pupils that have learned with me are some of the best judo men in the world today with forty years' experience; this means old people. Just like in Japan, the older they get, the better they get. It shows you that they have learned the real thing. Because Mifune fought twenty Japanese champions at the age of seventy-four publicly.

Let me ask you this: I want to know more or less what judo contributed to your current work.

Quite a lot, quite a lot.

In Body and Mature Behavior, *you talked about the position of the person's pelvis while standing or walking, and where the person's head is, and how it's compensated for, and the amount of fear they feel relative to such compensations ...*

Yes, yes. Well, first of all, that is actually in Kano, and I am sure that I meet Kano's views on that as closely as you can put it in the European language, that Japanese way of thinking. Kano and Koizumi, they always agreed with whatever formulation I made. The more we talked, the more we produced another way of putting it, a way sensible to the West.

Looking at Koizumi's book, he's an incredibly intelligent man. . . .

Oh, he is a marvelous ... look, in Japan they gave him eighth dan, though he really hadn't been in Japan for fifty years. He's a very learned and a very clever man and a very efficient man. Koizumi at the age of eighty could do that Five Winds kata thing [a unique way of sitting up, actually going from lying to standing and looking like it was done with the body straight.—DL.] that I taught you. And he was a national coach in Britain at the age of eighty, still being only one night a week at home, all the others traveling all over the place, greeting people, teaching, demonstrating, training, and instructing the higher-grade belts. It's very hard work, even for a young man. Koizumi has a little book on judo—have you seen it?

I have one.

Yeah, you see he throws Leggett,* and with Leggett demonstrates throws. Did you see that he has a little book of exercises? It's wonderful. In it you would see some of the things we do, like crossing and uncrossing the legs. You would see this old man open his legs just marvelously. Nobody here, none of the aikido experts can move as beautifully as he does, or get up with such soft movement. You can see it's a beautiful movement and you can see that he's half-naked, dressed only in shorts, so that you see the details of the movement. It's unbelievable because in the pictures, he's seventy-eight years old. The grace of the movement! A grace of the movement few dancers could achieve. And to photograph nude like that so that you see the movement, it's so marvelous, the whole body like one line. It's nice to see. I mean, even if you don't know what judo is you will just say, "Look, what a beautiful man, what a beautiful movement."

What was Kano's contribution to judo?

He created it.

What relation does it have to the older jujitsu?

---

*Trevor Leggett (1914–2000) was a legendary British judo man. He wrote more than thirty books on judo, Zen, and Japanese culture and was often referred to by Feldenkrais.

He took out of all of jujitsu those things ... You see, his idea was at that time ... that's a very interesting story in itself, how judo came to be. You know that the Americans came with the fleet into Japan with very strongly built sailors and marines and arriving in Japan where there were small little people. They were not all samurais. And those American chaps with their weight and strength and build made a terrific impression on the Japanese, so that they felt useless. The Japanese being separated from the world, they thought of themselves as being in the Land of the Rising Sun, as gods. They even have the rising sun on their flag today. And suddenly they found that some big, white idiots came around who were stronger and better fighters and could do anything to them. They were downhearted, the whole nation. And they tried by cleverness to cheat the Americans, to do anything to win. When they wanted to dispose of one, they would do it. But not by using strength but by strategy, and anything was permitted to get results. Because what can you do against an elephant who attacks you? What would you do? Would you consider it indecent to kick his balls? No, certainly not. So you kick his balls and that's that. You are proud of yourself that you did it, because if you didn't, you would be dead. And you know how karate came to be? MacArthur made it. General MacArthur produced karate.

You mean he is responsible for getting it to the West?

For getting it into Japan. Because, you see, judo had about five million active members in Japan. Counting those people who had done judo and stopped doing it, there were about ten million people who were involved in judo. And so MacArthur thought if they met in clubs, that's the kind of group of people that you could never hold down. Ten million people trained who can fight very efficiently. So the Japanese under the treaty were prohibited from practicing judo in Japan. General MacArthur prohibited judo in Japan. It was like the Communist Party, you can't meet together to do it. And so to people who were used to a lifetime of practice, for them it was a terrible thing. It was like taking a drunk and taking the bottle away from him. A person who is used to training three or four times a week, doing judo for a lifetime or ten, fifteen, twenty years, and who suddenly can't do it, has to do something. So, they started doing karate. They said, look, we won't do judo, or use the judo *gi* nor the judo mat, but we'll do *atemi* [striking]. *Atemi-waza*, only the hitting part. And that will help us actually to fight the Americans directly. And they started making out of that *atemi* an art. And so gradually all of Japan, all the sum of the judo people got into training again in this new thing which was not prohibited. So everybody practiced that instead of judo and therefore many, many people became involved in it. The skill of some of the judo men was actually put into karate and they evolved a spectacular fighting art where they could actually fight again with that same judo principle, but this time, that principle could not be avowed. It couldn't be called judo. Therefore, they did it in a different way so as to do a legal thing and not an illegal thing. For doing judo, they could be put in prison. And so gradually, karate became, in a few years with the American occupation of Japan, generally practiced in every club. Where every club had been a judo club, it became a karate club. So that's how it became what it is.

The other day when we were talking, you said that if you talked about ki, nobody would publish it, that they wouldn't want to hear about it. Right, you said that?

Mmmmm.

So my feeling is that I would like to talk about it anyway and . . .

It's not that I don't want to talk about it, but for me this starts with the organization of the body. To me, ki is not a thing and not a spirit and not an anything, but the way a body is organized to function and that way in which it functions best. It means that a body can produce with its weight, with the muscles that it has, with the brain it has, the greatest amount of work possible with a particular organization of that body, and that particular organization turns out to be central to the thing we're talking about. It's a complex appreciation of how a human body is made, how it functions: That it has a head that must not be involved in the movement but which must be free, whatever the movement is, to move anywhere; and that the lower abdomen must be in such a state that it can do all the things that it needs to do without disturbing the head. The rest of the body and the arms are not to be used to produce strength. And that is the truth. Once you get that, if you do, you can do judo throws, the most difficult ones; the heaviest person, you can throw him if you get that. But to the people who are keen on mysterious things of ki and chi, this is a complete comedown, and they are not interested. They don't want to listen to it. They don't want it to be like that.

It sounds like F. M. Alexander's* concept of "use" would be a more useful concept than that of ki.

Oh, no, that's not true because his "use" is a limited "use." With his use you can't throw anybody, you can't even throw yourself, you can't roll with that. So that's "use." Movement, motility, you can see, and my way of presenting chi was acceptable to Koizumi, a man whose movement was superb and effective until the age of eighty, being able to throw anybody, even if it was someone five times his own weight. He was pleased to think that chi's not a mysterious thing.

I am sure. So will a lot of people be pleased to hear that.

Yeah, and be able to learn to do it. It's not a question of either you have it or you don't.

What about equilibrium in relation to martial arts?

Oh, yes. The equilibrium of the martial arts is a very funny one. I can tell you, my mother is a frail, little woman and when she was eighty-four years

---

*F. M. Alexander (1869–1955) is the founder of the Alexander Technique, which has many theoretical overlaps with the *Feldenkrais Method*. Feldenkrais was influenced by his contact with Alexander and some of Alexander's main pupils during his stay in London. The term "use of self" was coined by Alexander to refer to one's overall state as one engages in life's activities. Alexander believed that unconscious habits often interfere with a good "use of self" and that conscious control was necessary to overcome these habitual tendencies.

old, she lifted me, with my weight, on her hip for a hip throw and it looked completely fake because it is just unbelievable. Because my mother is kind of . . . she probably inherited from me, a sort of mind like that. [Laughter] When she saw that people could do judo throws and lifts, she said, "I can do it," and it took her about ten minutes and she learned to do it. Everybody was watching because it seemed that she was really going to collapse under a weight like my own. She lifted my legs completely in the air, with the greatest ease, not making even the slightest effort of breath. I also have a picture of my sister lifting me and holding me up there. How did she get me there? I have the picture. That picture was published in France and was reproduced in about twenty different papers. Because it looked fake . . . a young girl, a little girl lifts a heavy, strong man and lifts him overhead like that in a way that only weightlifters can do—and not the average weightlifter could do it. How do you do that? You say it's done with ki, with chi. Now if I give you anything you want, buy some chi and ki and do it. Get some ki and chi from anybody you like and do it. Now the trick is this: the people who can do it say they have chi. That's the kind of . . . to me, that's exactly like saying my mother inherited it from me. It is putting the horse behind the cart.

So the equilibrium in the martial arts is a very peculiar, very strange one. You should be able to recover your equilibrium, your balance faster than the opponent and find any fault in his balance and take advantage of that. Now, how do you make your recovery faster than his? He's a human being and you're a human being and your loss of balance must be recovered faster than his, otherwise you cannot control him, and you certainly cannot do anything to him otherwise. Now, again, the general consensus is this: you do that because when you have chi, you can do it. Now I say, fuck yourself, and you can write it there. You can't do it unless you can do it. When you can do it, you can say you have ki. But to get it, you have to learn to organize yourself so that you can recover your balance faster than the opponent, and how do you do that?

Look at the way the eighth dan works with ordinary people or with a second or third dan. Do you see what happens? The chap destroys them and how does he do it? You can't even see it. Why is that? The lower dan attacks and nothing happens. The attacker may be vigorous and strong and noth-

154

ing happens. Why? Because the eighth dan recovers his balance first, and at the moment the other one attacks him, he is in complete control of his body and he changes and recovers his balance so fast that when the other one makes the slightest movement, he can take advantage of it. Now, the reaction time of people is approximately the same; the reaction time of the nervous system is similar from one person to another, within quite narrow limits unless the person is ill-formed. Therefore, what can be done, the recovery, the reorganization is only a way of linking that part of you which sees and hears and listens and feels. With your way of moving your pelvis and legs in order to be coordinated, there must be no waste of energy, no waste of work, no waste of push between the head and the spine and the pelvis. So that again shows you that there is an organization of bones and head, and the link between them is so organized that you can move fast. And when your organization is superior, then the reaction time is of no consequence. The neurological reaction time is the same for you as for him, but you organize yourself faster; therefore, you can recover balance faster than he can. Therefore, you beat him. And in judo, that's the thing that is really taught and done.

If you can compete for sixteen rounds it means you and your opponent are almost equal. And then if by chance one gets tired, you then get in a few bangs and win. I bet that if I present you a boy of ten, whether or not you know aikido or judo or anything, you will beat him in less than thirty seconds because you just lift him and throw him on the floor and break his neck. Therefore, when you are superior in strength, to that degree, there is no question of ki; you are just superior. A dog has very little trouble killing a cat if he only succeeds in getting him by the neck; one throw and the neck is broken. But you have never seen a cat destroying a dog. A cat can't do it. A cat will scratch out his eyes and that's what he does. When you neglect the weight, then the organization is the one and only thing that counts. When the body is organized so that you can move better and faster than your opponent, it's not a question of competing with him.

Kano showed that there are at least ten distinct grades of quality. Because a Mifune would never be beaten by a fifth dan, it's inconceivable. A Mifune would take a fifth dan and just throw him about but not compete with him.

The chap would say, "How did you do it?" and he would throw him again and again for about ten minutes and the chap would never know what was happening to him. Koizumi would throw fifty people like that, one after another, and they'd get up and ask how he did it. He'd say, "Look, I did it like this," and throw them again.

So you see, to me ki, like everything I do, is a concrete thing which can be taught and learned and which is common to every human being provided the man is willing to learn and he is a normal person, meaning he has no real defects. But even with defects, you can learn to do it.

[To Charles Alston] You can feel that when I threw you I was not pushing with a lot of strength, but somehow using your skeleton and the way you stand. To teach that, first you demonstrate putting too much into it, then too little, and then something in between. I could feel it. You can feel it. That's the kind of thing that I consider to be ki, that I can teach anybody. But if it is taught in a limited way, it will function only in that situation. To transfer that kind of limited learning to other things is a long job.

So you're saying that the mystical conception people carry around with them about ki is unnecessary. And that you don't need it.

I think that organization is necessary; otherwise you can't do it. But it is not a thing which—look, if ki were a spiritual quantity the way the psychic people may think, then suppose I have plenty of ki and I want to bestow you the ki. I somehow transfer to you some of the power, then you can do anything. You see? That's the idea. I think that idea is complete nonsense, but people like Kano have taught Mifunes and Nagaokas and Yokoyamas and all sorts of extraordinary people who were looked upon as godlike. That I can understand, and that I can teach you—not as well as Kano himself could, but not by half as much worse, because he is dead and I am alive. [Laughter]

So these organizations are hierarchical, and in the old days of Kano, the black belt was actually a designation of each order of organization. [psycho-neuro-muscular]

Oh, yes. I have the film that I told you about in which we have from first dan to the seventh. You can see that the difference is such that every time a higher grade goes against a lower grade, it looks incredible. The higher-ranked man who looked unbeatable and so fast against a lower grade than him when he goes against someone one grade higher than him, he is the underdog. That higher rank throws him as much as he wants every three seconds. Whatever the higher rank does, the other one falls. And whenever he falls, the higher rank holds him and does an arm lock, or strangles him, and can just do anything he likes, just like with a baby. And then this chap is, say, fourth dan, and here comes the fifth dan who makes out of him what? Just as if he wasn't there, again, throwing him, the one who looked unbeatable a little earlier, in the space of a minute, twenty, thirty times. He gets up and he's on the floor again. And the final dan, the seventh one, doing it to the sixth, that is a real extraordinary thing, because all the others do more or less work, but with these two, the seventh dan is doing it entirely in movement. He never stops to throw; he doesn't stop like they do nowadays, the silly asses, pushing each other. It never stops. He moves, moves around, and in the movement, he throws him. He never stops to do the throw. And that looks perfection itself, godlike. And the other chap can't do a thing. Now what can the other chap do? If he doesn't move, he gets thrown; so he moves. So they move all over the place, and each movement is a throw. Each movement is a throw. But on the tatami, they are in every corner. All the others throw somebody in the middle, but this seventh dan throws him in that corner, and that corner, in the middle, and there's always movement. And in a minute they go through about forty throws so fast that you don't know where they come from—you could see it afterwards in slow motion.

The question of what and how to produce change in the neuromuscular organization of a person and what it means to do so is a very difficult problem. You cannot examine the brain; you don't know what goes on in there. You can only judge the outward actions. Now in judo or in karate or in aikido, the problem is simple. The problem is only whether you have a good teacher or a bad teacher. A good teacher will prepare you. He will give you three opponents, for instance, for a first degree black belt grading test. The teacher will present the student with an orange belt, a blue belt, a green belt to beat and if he does that efficiently, not by mucking about three hours ... but if he in three minutes beats every one of the lower belts, which means he is superior to those people in skill, the teacher will take one brown belt, not one of the best, but a brown belt, and have the student try his skill. And if he can in a short time defeat this other brown belt too, then he will have no hesitation of promoting him. And the incredible thing that happens is that once he is promoted, the first time he puts on his black belt, he can beat any of those people that he previously had to compete with in a quarter of the time and do it regularly. The fact that he has been publicly acknowledged to have made the grade creates in him his own self-assurance. He has grown in his own eyes and he now has greater liberty to judge the opponent and see whether he can beat him or not. He doesn't compete anymore with those whom he previously had to struggle with. He beats them. So he must certainly be a higher grade. Now if the teacher is good, he brings the person to a level of skill and self-assurance so that when he puts him to the test, he has a great chance of succeeding. The bad teacher will just put him to the trial, in a contest, and if he is beaten by a blue belt or a green belt, it will take him another year or two before he can win a contest again with the same low-grade belts, because he is doubting his movement now. Therefore he is stiff, he is not free to move, his movements become much slower, much jerkier, too late, always hesitating. "Should I do it, shouldn't I do it? Is it a good time? I don't want to fail again"—like you saw Frazier in the last bouts he had. He lost though he was infinitely better than his opponent. He lost only because he was beaten before in earlier fights, because they knocked out of him the idea that he can win.

This is not a simple thing, the idea to win. You find that the fellow's movement becomes clumsy, that he misses opportunities, just because he is not free to look at his adversary. To beat somebody by skill, you must see when it can be done and when it can't be done. Skill doesn't mean that you force your head through the wall. Therefore, a good teacher will do this: Once he has tested the man successfully, he will teach him important things in the next few days because the man is free now to learn them. The teacher will teach the student things to make sure that he is never beaten by an inferior man. And how can he make sure? He will take a strong man and will tell this chap, this new black belt, to play with him and be taught how to escape. That means this strong chap will hold you and you learn how to get out. Therefore, the strong one doesn't really hold the chap full strength, and so he learns with somebody of whom he is really afraid. He becomes acquainted with him and sees how he could escape because he can see things which he couldn't before. After that the next time he will say, "Hold me seriously," and he will still get out. After that, the teacher will continue to guide him. Many of them become so beautiful to watch after they've been graded. Within the next week or two, they will beat people that have always beat them before. Those of the same grade who beat him before now can't do it. Now that is a new learning. He improves his skill to the point that in a year or nine months, the teacher can give him another trial, choosing the opponents for him with the likelihood that his skill will be effective and that he will beat them. And for the others who he beats, there will be no harm because they are supposed to be beaten by a higher grade. So to them it does no harm, but to him it does an immense power of good.

Therefore, you see, Kano was a very learned, clever man who organized that thing like that so that the real judo man can fight every real grade in the Kodokan. He is a master in his grade and people below his grade, he doesn't have to compete with, he just beats them. He can teach them. And therefore, he will let himself be thrown in order to teach them, because he knows he has nothing to defend. His honor is safe.

So, therefore, if your question is a particular question, about judo, aikido, and other things, you have your full answer. But if you want to see the general thing in, say, mathematics, then again it depends on the teacher. If the teacher is clever and he has taught you, say, matrices, he will present you a problem which, knowing what you have accomplished and how you learn, you are likely to solve. The solution will necessitate you being quiet, reposed, and relying on your skill of thinking. If he presents you with a problem above your head, you will fail, and the next year you will probably be one of the worst in the class, and a year later you will give it up altogether. You will say you are not [a] mathematician. If you have a teacher who wants you to learn, then you learn and grow, and grow all the time. If you have a teacher who wants to show you what a good teacher he is, he ruins most of the people. Only the one or two may succeed in spite of the bad teaching, but the rest of the class will be poor mathematicians. They won't be mathematicians. Now you can do that with everything. Therefore, when you talk about levels in the neurological way in the system itself, you know there are levels because they have been described by Jackson.* The spine can do all or nothing, no gradation. Therefore, you need the other centers, which will make this less jerky. The levels are hierarchical. And now that one level is attained the system will never stay there because once this level is good, you can achieve even better gradations, an even richer ...

Once you achieve a certain level, is it ever lost?

Oh, yes, it can be lost, always. That chap that has won a dan and you present him that same day with people with lower-grade belts that are stronger, better, and heavier than him, and if they beat him and if he is beaten four times running, he will go away from the club and never finish his training and think he is no bloody good. Any trauma, any task you or someone else puts to you above your ability will destroy you.

So that's there in everything, the neuromuscular levels. The hierarchies are as clear-cut developmentally as they are with a good teacher in judo or in kendo or in aikido or ... mathematics and physics.

---

*John Hughlings Jackson (1835–1911) was a seminal figure in nineteenth-century neurology. Here Feldenkrais refers to how Jackson conceived of the nervous system as having a hierarchical organization based on the organism's evolutionary history. Jackson delineated three centers in the brain going from lowest to highest. Lower corresponded to the earliest structures and higher referred to later arrivals such as the cortex, especially the prefrontal areas.

11

Moshe Feldenkrais Discusses Awareness and Consciousness with Aharon Katzir

Edited and with an Introduction by Carl Ginsburg

Carl Ginsburg, PhD, is one of Moshe Feldenkrais's original American students, and an active and respected teacher of the *Feldenkrais Method.* He has a wide background, including holding a doctorate in chemistry, making him well suited for editing this piece. Carl is also the editor of *The Master Moves,* a transcription of a workshop taught by Feldenkrais, and has written extensively on the Method. This article originally appeared in 2006, in *The Feldenkrais Journal.—Ed.*

Introduction

Moshe Feldenkrais, the conceiver and transmitter of the processes that became the *Feldenkrais Method,* wished to bring his innovative method and the ideas behind it to a wide public. As he synthesized and refined his work, he settled on the notion that the essence of what he was teaching and transmitting involved, above all, guiding his students to an improved sensory ability. The aim was to know one's self—how one can act and be effective in acting in daily life without self-interference and unexamined assumptions about the how of living. A keyword was "awareness. " The dialogue reproduced here was a major step in elucidating his intent. In this endeavor he chose to discuss the issues with his friend and biophysicist Aharon Katzir, also known as Katchalsky.

I became aware of Aharon Katchalsky some years ago while reading *Dynamic Patterns,* by J. A. Scott Kelso (published by MIT Press, 1995).

Professor Kelso noted that Katchalsky was a major figure in the early development of dynamic systems as a new way of understanding complexity in biology and particularly in the action of the nervous system. Kelso mentions that the agenda of dynamic systems was curtailed by the death of Aharon Katchalsky, who was slain by terrorists in Tel Aviv's Lod airport on May 30, 1972. A colleague then noted that Feldenkrais had mentioned a scientist friend who was killed in a terrorist raid. Aharon Katchalsky was indeed that friend.

In trying to trace down some information about Katzir and Feldenkrais in the ensuing years I found out about a tape of a conversation between Feldenkrais and Katzir in Hebrew that was made in the late '60s or early '70s. I found out that one of Feldenkrais's early students and now a trainer, Myriam Pfeffer, had a copy of that tape. She kindly helped arrange to have the contents of the tape transcribed and translated into English, and Michél Silice Feldenkrais, who headed the Feldenkrais Institute in Tel Aviv, kindly gave permission to have this transcript published. For that we can be very grateful because the material they discussed is more than of historic interest. Their theme lies at the very heart of Feldenkrais's search for an understanding of awareness.

The taped conversation recapitulates between the two participants their previous conversations in which they elucidated the essence of "awareness" as each understood the term. Dr. Katzir contributes from his background in biophysics, Dr. Feldenkrais from his investigations, which led to the development of his *Method*. The conversation is truly a dialogue, and through the interplay of ideas and conceptions a new view of awareness comes into focus. They start with describing their own beginning ideas. The evolving discussion leads to reformulations and clarifications. As you read the dialogue, be aware that this is a conversation between two curious thinkers and that the result of their process does not become clear until the end. This final result is a stunning statement of the intentions of Dr. Feldenkrais in developing the work that has been passed down to his successors, and defines awareness as an evolutionary step for humankind. It is worth the struggle to follow the process.

I have edited the transcript for clarity and smoothness and eliminated repetitions. I have also tried to make sure that what was difficult to translate is coherent in the context of understanding the thoughts expressed. In this I have taken editorial liberties to be accurate to the thinking of the two participants rather than to stay within the bounds of a literal translation. Where words and phrases were often incomplete, I have filled in for continuity and clarity of the text. These additions are indicated by [brackets] surrounding the added material. I have also included some [endnotes] to help clarify the discussion.

I thank Ravhon Niv for his transcription and translation from the Hebrew, which proved to be a challenging task, and Chava Shelhav, an early student of Feldenkrais and a trainer, for checking the accuracy of the transcript.
—Carl Ginsburg

MOSHE FELDENKRAIS: I don't remember how we decided that consciousness and awareness without action is impossible. You say that you remember the pathway. Would you try then to evoke the main stages?

AHARON KATZIR: I wish to bring back our way of discussion. Our point of departure was "What is an absolute knowledge?" I think we asked ourselves what is the potency of one sentence. And then I claimed in one argument that the certain knowledge is composed of two elements: the concepts and the correlation of concepts. The elementary concepts are perceptible concepts, certain images that come in via our sense organs to our consciousness and are joined in our consciousness into elements of knowledge. I accept these elements as certain after they have become a concept. Maybe you remember, we were talking about how sensation can be variable. I can see something as red in one moment, yet in a different light I can see it as yellow or colorless or as black. But after the concept of red is formed in my mind, then the red is a certainty even at the moment the red image changes with a sensational alteration.

Yes, we agreed that certainty is our capacity to assemble the concepts with the help of laws, what we call the laws of logic. These laws might change, for instance, under the impact of science, such as the law of causality. But in one sense of [thinking], in a certain time period I assemble the concepts [until I have] a certain lawfulness and rightfulness. The lawfulness becomes certain for me just as the concept itself. I can say that concepts are then assembled [into] sentences.

We accepted that what is true in knowledge are the concepts and the lawful correlations of concepts. But then you claimed that knowledge itself is not the same as awareness, not part of a [true] human reality. You spoke of knowledge that is dead—for example, the knowledge buried in books. We can have a library full of knowledge, but we cannot consider it as awareness. And so you brought as an example of this distinction, and I believe a good one, that I can come across this chair millions of times and I have an impression of it, and yet I don't have awareness. That is because if you ask me how many slats there are in the back of this chair, I may not be able to answer. On the other hand, if I concentrate my mind to rebuild its image and then answer you as to how many slats comprise the back of the chair, we have another element, but a very important one. This element turns consciousness into awareness.

FELDENKRAIS: We can add here something that might not be very important. In a hypnotic state we can recall this information. Thus this information was registered by part of the mind, but if the awareness was not modified during the recording of it, it cannot be restored to consciousness.

KATZIR: And then I brought an example: Gurdjieff's[1] claim that our consciousness resembles very much a sleep state in which I absorb many things which do not become consciously fixed, and in which [my attention] jumps from one place to another. If a person tries seriously to measure for how long he concentrates on one fact, he finds out that it doesn't last very long. [Attention] jumps from one topic image to another. Awareness, on the other hand, is a process of full concentration, a process of clear analytic action on the points you deal with at that particular moment.

That brought us to think that the difference between consciousness and awareness is in [operational concepts]. Consciousness is a collection of images organized in a certain manner into something that resembles a mechanical operation. Awareness is higher and freer, involving a real [use of an operational procedure]. And then we agreed that the difference between awareness and consciousness is the principle of activity.

Afterwards we checked this question: What is the substance of an operation? On the one hand, people like Bridgman[2] claim that the great discovery of science is that every concept involves an operation that can be carried out. Einstein's greatest insight is that in physics there is no meaning to concepts which are not operational. For example, he put in place of the common notion of time, which stands outside of physics [that is, a time existing as an absolute time-frame], a notion of time which is integrated into physics, as it is measured by [an instrument such as] a clock. It is [as if time is] thus inside the clock. The clock does not measure something objective, absolute, but time is [defined by] the clock. And therefore, if I cannot correlate clocks I cannot correlate times. The relativity of time results from the relativity of its measurement. The same is true for distance measurements.[3]

However, we arrived at the conclusion that Bridgman's concept of an operation is too narrow and that we cannot get very far with it. There are too many concepts that Bridgman would reject, and would claim that these do not exist. He says, for example, "For me God does not exist because I don't know what is the physical operation needed to measure God." But we arrived at the conclusion that this is a kind of narrowness, a useless limitation. I do not have a specific operation to measure wisdom or goodness. Nevertheless, in the aesthetic world, in the moral world, it is very easy for me to know [what is good and what is wise], although I do not have a physical operation for measuring, or let's say an operational system for this purpose.

Bridgman takes as another point a fictitious operation, which he calls "the paper and pencil operation." Whatever he can put on a paper is also an operation. Of course the whole thing is attained verbally. I can symbolically put it on the paper, but then the content of this fictitious operation will be lost, too. On the other hand, we introduced the notion of the mental operation that distinguishes awareness from consciousness. Moreover, we said that this operation involves the mind-body. Here is Bridgman's real mistake. He thought that every operation must involve movement that you can see, such as that of the hands and legs. But we said that the mental operation, the one that [indicates awareness], not necessarily the conscious one, is also manifest in an operation of the muscles. It manifests itself as very small changes that can be measured only with very sensitive methods.

FELDENKRAIS: I want to add something on this issue in order to confirm your last words. Many physiologists and those who work with electronic machines have dealt with this issue: How do we recognize something as a square? When a square is close to the eye it has one form and when it is far away a different form altogether. When it stands diagonally we can still recognize it as a square. How does the eye and the brain recognize the square? I found out by myself by training my awareness to notice how it depends mainly on the movement of the eyes. If you check yourself, you will see that when you think of a square, the eyes do the movement of a right angle four times. Try to think of a square and if you learn to listen to your eye movements, you will clearly feel that the eyes make the movement with the four angles. Because this movement is very precise you slowly learn to sense the eyes' movement as a square while you think of a square.

I remember that at this moment in our discussion, we started to talk about the difference between the external world and the internal world as a superficial distinction and one that depends on our short sight. Actually, our nervous system receives information from the outside through the eyes, the ears, and the nose, and from the body itself through the interoceptive nerve endings, what we call proprioception. In the moment of perceiving, our brain differentiates among the inputs which were received this way, and recognizes those inputs it received from the eyes, ears, and nose as external information. However, in actuality, our nervous system does not have a direct relation to the outside world, but always reads whatever was registered inside the body on the sensory level.[4]

Here I think you remarked that even this difference of inside and outside blurs when we look at it closely, because we sense heat in our skin, in our bones, even though the heat source can be at a distance, and not in direct contact. Then we cannot discern [at the sensory level] that it does not come from the body itself but rather from the surroundings. So in fact, theoretically we can say that the nervous system does not have a direct connection with the outside world. The distinction is completely artificial [an artifact of the nervous system itself].

KATZIR: I am glad that you brought up the problem of the objective and the subjective. The subjective part is the part from the reception of the sensation until the conscious reception; this is the subjective world. The aware image is the beginning of objectivity. After all, the objective also is inside ourselves, an integral part of ourselves exactly like the subjective, and the capacity to be aware is the objective within the subjective. The instrument that objectifies the subjective is the one which enables a human being to uplift one's self. And from this point of view the instrument of awareness is an instrument of freedom for the human being. As long as the human being is attached to the subjective, one is completely taken by the sensation and its conscious image. Without it being processed by awareness, a person is enslaved and bound.

Awareness then frees the human being in the sense that it turns his concepts to objectives. Therefore, developing awareness is increasing man's objectivity in order to liberate him from the limitations accompanied by subjectivity. We both agreed that Gurdjieff is correct in saying that developing awareness, the capacity to concentrate and the capacity to analyze, enables one to stand above one's own sense of limited subjectivity and unites one to a higher unity; it frees one from personal ambitions and from centering one's attention exclusively on oneself as his own subject. This enables awareness to stand beyond or above the "I" and to look at this "I" from the outside.

FELDENKRAIS: At this moment we found it necessary to find what we mean when we refer to awareness. We need to find something much more perceptible, much more pragmatic, on which we can have an influence.

I claimed that awareness is that part of the thinking mechanism that listens to the self while I am acting. We kept on looking for the foundation of awareness. Where is it? In which part of the system can we find it?

We debated for a long time this question. [I made this argument:] At the moment a person loses consciousness, what does he lose? First of all he loses orientation. For example, every person when he comes back to consciousness, the first thing he asks is "Where am I?" That is to say, at that moment he ceases to know where he is, he ceases to know that he is thinking, breathing, lying down, and so forth. And it continues. He can remember, for example, if he had been hit, that the rest of the essential mechanisms can be working—but not the awareness. He does not know "where he is." It seems to me very important because it opens a doorway as to where to look. Actually I have a whole range of phenomena which enable me to follow awareness and open the way to developing it.

I also asked you if it has ever happened to you that you fell asleep and changed your position while sleeping so that when you woke up you could not recognize at first where the door was or where the ceiling was. And I asked if at that moment you felt a kind of fear. Or it may happen that you have fainted partially, and did not know how. You find then no possibility to control your thinking.

You told me it has never happened to you. Personally it has happened to me. I remember clearly that several times in my life I woke up in a direction in which, at first, I did not know where is the head, where is the door, where is up or down. I found myself suspended, head downward, and at that moment, I knew very clearly that I could not recognize where I was. I could not do any movement until I adapted myself while opening my eyes, and came back to the more-or-less normal position of the head relative to space. At that moment immediately I was back in control. In other words, I regained the awareness of where I was, what I was doing, and where all this happened. I do not remember what you said about that.

KATZIR: As a matter of fact, the conclusion deriving from your model that I absolutely agree with is the following: the awareness functions in categories very similar to the Cartesian categories, and these categories are not absolute, as your demonstrations revealed, but categories of the awareness itself. And when the awareness in some of its parts is blurred and its categories cannot work, the conception of our world cannot exist.

What you told about orientation fits precisely the aware categories of space. These are like the Cartesian categories of space. Here it was revealed very clearly that the spatial category [perception] is not absolute. Only when the moment of awareness would arise, would you [be oriented] in the absolute [physical] space. Thus it became clear that our category of space is psychological and can be changed by interaction with [what] science [tells us]. If science will change its spatial category then our psychological categories will change, too. But here you really brought up the first spatial category, the psycho-physiological data, what is on the edge of the psychological and physiological data of space. That a psychological state which modifies the organs of equilibrium and modifies the conception [perception) of space [exists], makes it so that you cannot use the data of awareness to create an image out of them. This is so until you create for yourself the spatial category.

Here is an example: Through experiments with chemicals like mescaline we can modify the category of time and then the whole time conception of our life and the order of the aware data in time changes radically. A person who is under the influence of mescaline will be in a state like your example of waking up out of sleep without having an orientation of space. A person under the influence of mescaline is not situated in the normal dimension of time, but in a very different one. We can hypothetically imagine that if we could go to the origins of psycho-physiological categories, we would remove the whole philosophical fog about the absolute and of eternity, and that the operative-aware [experiential] origins of the deep foundation of philosophy would reveal themselves.

FELDENKRAIS: I have no doubt about it. Let us continue with the subject of awareness, the orientation. First of all, this connection in itself enables the possibility for clear research on the development of awareness. This is because the development of awareness and orientation goes hand in hand. The child from the beginning does not understand what is up or down. It is clear then that awareness is something that grows with the child. It develops and is not given from birth. In that case, it is controllable and because it is learned it can be learned again. We can find out if the learning is done properly.

I think the learning of awareness in most people is stopped much too soon. Many of the scientists think that the human brain develops fully by the age of fourteen, that the intelligence developed by the age of fourteen is stable. It won't grow any further. I think that is not fully true because by the age of fourteen we keep on developing our orientation capacities and the body's characters and traits in gravity. Afterwards we neglect it. The one who neglects the improvement of his own understanding stops the improvement of awareness at the same time. We can, of course, do something with those elements, something experimental or something we can go with. But I developed this knowledge in a much more profound manner. But of course in our first conversation we touched only the rudiments. I give the floor over now to you.

KATZIR: At this point I wanted to remind ourselves, what were the questions that we asked ourselves? Are the categories of our awareness permanent and unchangeable? Even if science obliges us to a change of categories, is our awareness capable of adjusting itself? We came to the conclusion that our categories are not arbitrary but verbal and therefore we can imagine an evolution of the categories of awareness adjusted to the dynamic of awareness itself.

This is because science in the first place enlarges awareness and [creates] new facts on the basis of the expanded awareness. The problem is how to adjust awareness to consciousness. For example, until the "I" is registered in the human being and becomes an integral part of his life, a person cannot accept a relative world. Until then our awareness should be Euclidean and Platonic,[5] whereas the experience to adjust our awareness to a relatively tolerant world, which gives equal rights to all relation systems, to all coordination systems, is something that requires the same kind of revolution as the Copernican revolution.

Or as another example, we have the principle of uncertainty[6] and the renunciation of absolute causality and the willingness to see variable causes instead of monovalent causes, causes from the domain of modern physics. According to the dynamic conception, the evolution of categories themselves suggests that there is hope that man will be able to change the categories of his mind and soul. And out of this, a very important conclusion: It is true that from the physiological and biological aspects man has gone through very small changes in the structure of his body during the last fifty thousand years—that is to say, from the creation of *Homo sapiens*. Considering only the coarse physical aspect, the changes have been apparently small. On the other hand, the impression we have is that awareness has gone through an enormous evolution during these last fifty thousand years. There is no doubt, though, that the conscious ability, the elementary conceptual ability, of the *Homo sapiens* twenty thousand years ago and today was very much alike. On the other hand, there is no doubt that awareness following consciousness has gone through decisive changes. In that case, when we talk about evolution, we talk about the evolution of awareness, and we can even think of the basic direction of evolution is of awareness, a consolidation of man's orientation, the continual evolution of man's categories, a continuation of concentration, and the creation of free objectivity. This last is the path perhaps to what we can call maturity, in the sense of the human being rising above himself, becoming the objective person who sees himself from a higher distance and can develop without stopping, without limit. Within the limited frame, the unchanging physical basis, the awareness does not have any limits to its development.

FELDENKRAIS: And I agreed with what you said, and I can see very clearly that in our awareness we see a very small part of the possible orientation of our body. Most people, for example, look only to the front and to the sides but very few look up and down. And most of us do not pay attention; we do not look at ourselves, do not pay attention to others or to other organs. If we try to check ourselves we find afterwards that many parts of the body, in fact most of the body, is not there; the person does not listen to himself in his awareness while acting. This is one of the major things for awareness: to connect that which is perceptible, the impressions that are received. We can then supervise the way in which it is recorded in the body. Let us take a simple example: I am walking down the street where I pass every day and ask myself, How many windows are there in the building next to me? Although I may have seen the building a thousand times I cannot tell. But if I go once with the intention to see how I can remember, while I know what I am doing, a part of my attention is directed to myself while I am acting and looking and thinking of what I see. And then I can see with such a clarity that I absorb the clarity, and come back home and see things in a new way. And this happens even though I saw the same things thousands of times without noticing anything.

KATZIR: You justly remarked that we use our awareness for only a very small part of the options we have. We agreed on much less than one percent, perhaps not even one thousandth part. By the way, this remark reminds me of the well-known observation about the physiology of the brain, that in the gray membrane of the big brain, huge areas are empty and unexploited. Only very small parts of the gray membrane are connected with a function; a huge area is "blank." That is an immense potential you can fill with awareness, which at the moment does not exist.[7]

In addition to this we discussed the topic of developing a free awareness that enables a critical and free operation which results from the needs of self-awareness. From a certain point of view, we can think of this as a process of de-conditioning—that is to say, "un-conditioning." And then we talked about the culture, which is stipulated by the possibility of conditioning. Because without conditioning there can be no language, there can be no mutual understanding among people. No valid social concepts can exist. No behavior could exist either. Not only from the social communication point of view, but no behavior could exist particularly in a technocratic society in which all its actions are stipulated by your ability to impose on yourself a system of conditioned reflexes that enable you to live. But along with that we know that the actual conditioning caused a delay in the development of awareness and also created "blanks" of enormous area that could be used freely by now.[8]

Therefore, the big problem is the problem of harmony between the conditioned area which was determined by social needs, and the de-conditioning, the liberation in which we develop a self-active part which liberates the individual from his subjective enslavement. We talked about some of the schools of the Far East, such as Zen Buddhism or certain schools of yoga, which are attempts at de-conditioning while preserving a minimum of conditioning that enables man to stay in society.

FELDENKRAIS: I marvel at your memory and your capacity to renew the whole issue about which we talked the other time, but I think you skipped one topic. I think it was like this: I mentioned Professor Guthrie[9] and his theory of learning, and said that he is to my opinion the only psychologist who understands the issue of creating concepts and behavior and placing it absolutely with muscles and action. According to him, no action in the world, no thought, no feeling, is independent of muscle mobility, in the sense of a conditioned response in each action. In his opinion everything is being accomplished in each action. Every action is absolute conditioning exactly as if it is done within the limit of the hands of time. That is to say, the unconditioned reaction ..., the conditioned stimulus ..., the conditioned reflex ..., I am confusing everything. If the stimulus arouses a conditioned reflex, it must be approximately within the limit of three seconds. According to Pavlov's conditioning experiments, fifty repetitions are needed to get the maximum [learning] from this phenomenon. But these experiments were with dogs. With people, according to Guthrie, every action is a phenomenon of conditioning [association] but because the action is repetitive, the next action can be done with an opposite conditioning [association] so that gradually we lose the capacity to follow the way of learning.[10] [On the other hand,] if the repetition is in a clear direction when the conditioning is accomplished and this is the ability ... this is learning. But it is impossible to know in advance whether this action of conditioning will do the action of learning or not. It is a matter of fortuitousness, of chance. We can see only afterwards. I think that after this you said what you said before.

KATZIR: Maybe I will complete your words. Learning is a very complicated system. The attempt to generalize the learning process in a simple phrase like "Learning is conditioning" is without any doubt only a partial truth. It is certain that a big part of the very elementary part of learning is conditioning. In order to teach a person to walk, you need to create a whole system of conditioned reflexes that will make the legs function harmoniously with the movement of the hands, the eyes, and so on. But even the elementary learning includes a higher conditioning. The founder of cybernetics, Norbert Wiener, claimed that one of the elements of learning at a higher level is the ability to correct on the basis of feedback. In a machine run by a conditioned reflex, an impression is received, transmitted then to a coordination center, and an operation results in a fixed trajectory. But the sophisticated modern machine has a feedback instrument that receives information from the outer world and corrects the operation ceaselessly. So if the operation does not lead to the intentional result and purpose, it corrects itself. Thus even elementary education is not conditioning—namely, a creation of fixed trajectories and tracks—but also the ability to correct them ceaselessly. In other words, above the track of conditioning there is always a possible track of de-conditioning and of creation of new tracks and trajectories. When you put awareness to the elements, you become sensitive so that you can shift the elements.

FELDENKRAIS: Since you mentioned at the last moment the word *awareness*, I have almost nothing to add. Yet this is exactly what I wanted to say. The last time we talked lengthily to establish that as long as there is no awareness the conditioning is completely automatic. Only through feedback can an action become a new habit in life, or at the contrary be rejected. But this is possible only through the light of awareness. Because awareness is a part of the correction, it is turned into the action itself; it listens to the action. Such listening, I think, is the first feedback. In other words, without feedback it is impossible to condition or de-condition a grown-up person. This awareness is, as a matter of fact, what cybernetics requires as feedback. All servo-mechanisms[11] require feedback. And when we look at our system, we find that it is made of thousands of feedbacks.

When I look with my eyes at a book and read and I don't read the whole page ... and I don't know what I read either, then I go over it again and ask, what is different at that moment? At that moment I listen to myself and to what I read. In other words, I use feedback and therefore I read in a new manner, in a new light. So I can clearly see what I see, I can see what I know and understand—and even what I did not understand.

KATZIR: But there is something more and it is the important thing, in my opinion. We must distinguish between human awareness and the automatic servo-mechanism in the sense of cybernetics. Mechanical feedback brings back the image to a ready-made schema and corrects the operation according to this schema. That is to say, in every servo-mechanism, in every automatic mechanism a fundamental pattern is installed which guides, corrects, and directs the whole thing. The uniqueness of awareness is its ability to create schemas. And perhaps the creating of schemas is the act of creation itself. In other words, if we ask what creation is, perhaps the deep content of the notion of creation is the ability to construct new schemas.

FELDENKRAIS: That is completely true, yet I can confirm it only in my own way, which is this: The awareness of most people is so undeveloped, so poor, that the moment a person sees a new phenomenon, he puts it in a pattern or a schema like a machine. He relates it and compares it with the traits and qualities he already knows as if he refuses to look at it as a new thing. That is to say, he makes no self-observation. How do you say it in Hebrew? Self-examination is not possible, is not done. In fact, it is an illusion if the person, while he is listening, while he is thinking and looking, he is judging at the same time, saying, "This is good," "This is not good," "That's it," "That is not it." At this precise moment he interrupts the ability of his awareness to see clearly and correctly. If we observe a little child while his awareness is developing, we can see that when he sees an unfamiliar object, he will usually look at it and does not judge, does not compare. We can observe that he becomes silent. He does not hear and does not see anything else. It is impossible to divert his attention; he just looks and sees what he sees. And that attracts his whole attention. Of course, as we said, it is the ability to observe while he is listening to himself. He does not have any other attention. All his awareness is drowned in it. We can observe this ability only in children or in those who kept this childish virtue, some of whom we call erudite, learned people. That childish virtue is namely the ability to look at something without preparing the fixed mechanical feedback, but instead to illuminate what is found, to light it up in our awareness, to let the mechanism be nourished and sated by it without any prior deliberation and judgment. This is the clearest ability of awareness that we are able to achieve up to now. And I think this ability can be learned and directed to the extent that it will not be a rare moment in the life of human beings. We can make it something systematic, a state which we can learn and use most of the time.

KATZIR: To your last words there are two points to add. Let's go back for a while to the subject of human creativity, where we came to the conclusion that man needs creativity. Erich Fromm described it in his book *The Sane Society*. He wrote that the social illness of the modern, developed, capitalistic regime is the loss of the ability, the capacity, of the modern man to create. If we refer to what we said before—that modern man must adjust his operations to one general schema[12] in which he does not participate, and did take part in its processing [organization]—[we can agree with] Erich Fromm that modern man is handicapped in his aware function by the deprivation of his higher function of creating schemas, which is the highest manifestation of creation. This is what is lost. We can continue from there to the second direction you mentioned, the creation of new schemas. It is not conditioning, because conditioning is a fixed track and not [the same as those] combinations that are the essence of those new schemas. We said the act of creation requires lability [flexibility], contrary to the rigid stability of the conditioning schema.

Therefore, the problem we are talking about is actually a different expression of something common, the preservation of the labile system, which enables an infinity of new combinations, which we will call the schemas of a creative pattern. This mental lability, which is the condition for creation, allows for free observation and new combinations taken from these unbiased and unconditioned observations. From this point of view the un-conditioning takes place by itself using the data which come to you from the external world.

FELDENKRAIS: As much as I can remember, we actually had spoken about reversibility, which is connected organically to lability. We spoke about Freud's model of a rope, darkness, and a window, yes, of the unconscious and the conscious and I claimed that one of health's dimensions is the ability to listen through the window to the room at such a speed and at such an ease that those two things are always connected together in action.

But right now we do not have patience anymore. We want to listen to what we have been saying.

12

Movement and the Mind

Interview with Will Schutz

Will Schutz, PhD (1925–2002) was a practicing psychologist who taught at Tufts University and Harvard University and made important contributions to his field. In the 1960s he moved his practice to Esalen Institute, a famous center for personal growth and human potential located on the California coast. He was the author of a number of books, including *Joy: Expanding Human Awareness* (1967) and *Profound Simplicity* (1979). Dr. Schutz learned of Moshe Feldenkrais's work in Israel and visited him there in the late '60s. He became an important sponsor and supporter of Feldenkrais and was responsible for Feldenkrais's first extensive teaching trip[1] to the United States in 1972, when Feldenkrais came to Esalen and taught a month-long course. This piece is based on a discussion/interview between Schutz and Feldenkrais in 1976, for the New Dimensions Radio program, a popular ongoing show devoted to alternative perspectives and holistic health.—*Ed.*

MOSHE FELDENKRAIS: Life is movement. If we act, if we move, we exist. If we don't move, we are dead. Therefore, a body that doesn't move is not a living thing. However, a living body cannot move by itself. In fact, if we made up a body with the best skeleton available and the finest muscles we could find, and we put them together, we would see that a dumb thing like that wouldn't be able to stand on its feet for a millionth of a second. It would fall because it had no brain. So the brain and the mind are just as much a part of our material structure as the bones and muscles.

Now, the functioning of the brain is quite different from the functioning of the skeleton and the other parts of the material structure. Structure and function must go together in any living thing. The most important aspect of functioning is what the mind does, what the brain does. Who has ever seen a mind without a brain? The brain is the material support of the mind, just as the body is the material support of the brain.

Suppose we make a machine that incorporates a skeleton, muscles, organs, and also a brain. Would a brain like that speak English or Turkish? It wouldn't know how to speak at all. Would a brain like that be able to read, to think mathematics, to listen to or create music? Could it make an IBM machine or a microphone? Of course not. When the brain comes into the world, it is fit to do only what any animal brain can do: it attends to breathing, to digestion, to the automatic processes of the body. Beyond that, we must "wire-in" that brain to relate to the environment into which it comes. At the outset, the brain doesn't even know how to stand. It cannot read or whistle, or tap dance, or skate, or swim. The brain must be adjusted and connected in order to fully function.

Assume I'm looking at a microphone. When my eyes look at it, I identify the image. Actually, there is no image of a microphone in my brain. There is an image of the microphone on my retina. However, from the retina, the image from each eye is separated into two parts and projected on four different parts of the cerebral cortex, which actually has no real image of a microphone. However, the function of seeing evokes in my mind the thing that I see with my eyes. The brain goes through a type of schooling that "wires" it in to objective reality. Reality, therefore, encompasses the environment and the body itself.

For instance, a baby cannot interlace the fingers until the first year has passed. Each child born must explore and learn his or her own body. The mind gradually develops and begins to program the functioning of the brain. My way of looking at the mind and body involves a subtle method of "rewiring" the structure of the entire human being to be functionally well-integrated, which means being able to do what the individual wants. Each individual has the choice to wire the body in a special way. However, the way we do it now is almost completely futile, making everyone alienated from their own capacity to have feelings.

The most important thing is not that we learn, but how we learn. After we are born, what language do we begin to speak? Naturally, it is the language that is spoken where we are born. Therefore, we're wired-in by that accident of birth, not by our choice, not by our capacities, not by our talents. Each language embodies cultural traditions and attitudes from thousands of years of development. Consequently, that language wires in to us a lot of notions which we don't want, which we accept merely because of learning the language. We learn a lot of old nonsense which perpetuates itself. Obviously, then, when we do learn, we can learn things wrongly.

Each person is born as a humanoid, a human animal. The newborn baby can swallow, suck, digest, excrete, and maintain body temperature like any other animal. What makes us different from animals is that humanoids can develop into *Homo sapiens,* human beings with intelligence, knowledge, and awareness.

WILL SCHUTZ: Your method is what I would call a self-oriented method, as opposed to a guru-oriented method. When I was doing some of your lessons, one particular example stood out. The problem was how to put my feet apart so that they were most comfortable. You told me to put them very close together and feel what that felt like, then put them very far apart and see what that felt like, and keep moving them back and forth until it felt right. Whatever felt right, was right, was correct. At that same time I was also going through Arica training, which I consider a guru-oriented approach. Oscar Ichazo[2] is the guru, and followers do what he says. I was doing a similar movement there, but the rule there was that you put your feet one forearm-length apart. If you didn't do that, then the instructor would come along and say, "That's not right. You didn't get it correct." What was "right" there depended on remembering what I was told to do by the instructor, rather than on what felt right to me.

MOSHE FELDENKRAIS: I never force anyone to accept my view. I would never say "This is correct" or "This is incorrect." To me there is nothing correct. However, if you do something, and don't know what you are doing, it's incorrect, for you. If you do know what you are doing, then whatever you do, you are correct. As human beings we have the peculiar ability, which other animals do not have, to know what we are doing. That's why we have freedom of choice.

Suppose I see you placing your feet apart at a distance which I consider incorrect. Now, why do I consider it incorrect? Not because I think it should be a certain length, but because I feel that you are really uncomfortable and are standing that way only because you have never actually visualized what distance is necessary in order to feel comfortable. You're not really concerned with whether it's comfortable or not. If you're very shy or if you are a virginal girl, you hold your feet together because it's prescribed to be "decent." If you are a show-off extrovert, wanting to show how important and free you are, you will open your legs much too wide. Much too wide for whom? Not for me. I don't say "This is right" and "This is wrong." I say that if you know that you are holding your feet close because you are shy, and you feel awkward spreading them, there is no harm. From my point of view, it's correct; do what you like. I am not here to tell you what to do. I am here only to show you that you should do what you know you are doing. However, if you don't really know that you hold your feet like that, and you believe that all human beings should hold their feet together, and you are virtually unable to open them, not because your physiology or your anatomy doesn't permit it, but because you are so unaware that you don't know that they can be opened, then it's incorrect.

WILL SCHUTZ: I remember an example, in one of the lessons I took with you, where that was illustrated. We were following some instructions, and one person in our class would not do it the way you said. Rather than bawl him out, you asked the rest of the class to do it the way he did it, then do it the way you said to do it, and to judge for ourselves which way was more comfortable. The process helped us to increase our awareness of what actually felt better.

MOSHE FELDENKRAIS: There's more to it than that. My point was that I said something, and the great majority of people did it in one way. There was one who somehow interpreted the same words quite differently. Now, it's possible that he is an idiot, that he can't understand what I'm talking

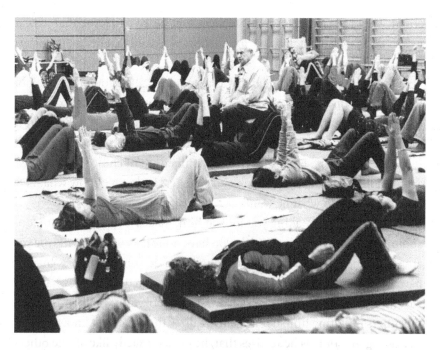

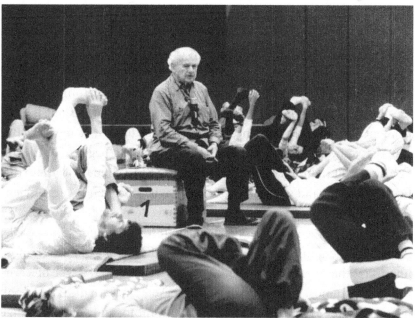

Seminar in 1981, Freiburg in Breisgau, Germany.

about. That's all right. However, I believe that he isn't an idiot, that instead he's so far away from being able to function as I asked that he can't conceive that I meant what I said.

Now, all the other people did it as asked. I tell all of them, "Look, look how this person does it. Maybe he is right; perhaps it should be done like that. Can you imitate him?" Yes, everybody can. "Can you do it the way you did before?" Yes, they all can, but he can only do it in his way; he cannot do it like all the others. Hence they have the freedom of choice between two acts, but he is a compulsive, unable to change. He doesn't know what he is doing; he can't do what he wants.

That technique, making you look at him, makes it easy for him to look at himself. I can say to him, "Look, you have done it as you have. Maybe you are right. These people can do like you, or can do something else, but you have no choice. You are a computer; they are human beings. They have free will; they have choice. You haven't. Now, sit and look. Can you see?" By seeing the others imitating him, he suddenly realizes that he didn't know what he was doing. As soon as he realizes that, he does it exactly like all the others. His learning takes ten seconds. He recaptures his freedom of choice and regains human dignity.

Understand that there are two sorts of learning. There is the kind of learning which is committing things to memory—for instance, taking a telephone book and learning it by heart, or taking an anatomy book and learning the attachments and origins of each muscle. That learning is independent of time and experience. You can decide to do it at any time. But suppose you want to play the piano. Every time you begin to learn, you say, "Look, all right, I haven't played the piano as a child. Now it's so difficult to start it, and what's the point of playing the piano? I am a scientist; I am a radio interviewer. What do I have to play the piano for? If I need a piano, somebody plays the piano on records." But for some people, like Yehudi Menuhin or Vladimir Horowitz,[3] the making of music is more important than your radio or your science. They learn by a type of learning which is almost beyond personal choice. You can learn the phone book if you want to, or not learn it if you don't want to; and you can change your mind.

184

But there is a learning in which you have no say whatsoever, and that learning is latent in the natural laws which have produced our brain and our nervous system and our body and our muscles. These laws are included in the cosmic laws of the universe. They are so precise and so sequential that you have no say about the order you will learn them in. They must be learned in that order; if not, you will not develop as a normal human being. You will be a cripple or an autistic child—something not normal. Why can't you teach a baby even a year old to hold a pencil and write? The baby cannot write until the capacity develops.

You see, there is a kind of learning which goes with growth. You cannot skate before you can walk, no matter how clever you are, even if you are a genius. You must first learn to walk. You cannot walk before you crawl. If you learn to walk before you crawl, you will be a cripple. You cannot learn to speak before you are vertical. You know why you can't? In the human nervous system, each part comes into function in a sequence, one after another. The functioning helps the growth at each stage as a new part of this brain comes into dominance, and changes the entire way of action. This type of learning must proceed at its own pace. We have no say in it. However, because this learning is done under human direction, it may be done in a different way than was intended by nature.

My way of learning, my way of dealing with people, is to find out, for that person who wants it, what sort of accomplishment is possible for that person. People can learn to move and walk and stand differently, but they have given up because they think it's too late now, that the growth process has been completed, that they can't learn something new, that they don't have the time or ability. You don't have to go back to being a baby in order to function properly. You can, at any time of your life, rewire yourself, provided I can convince you that there is nothing permanent or compulsive in your system, except what you believe to be so.

I don't treat patients. I give lessons to help a person learn about himself or herself. Learning comes by the experience of the manipulation. I don't treat people, I don't cure people, and I don't teach people. I tell them stories, because I believe that learning is the most important thing for a human being. Learning should be a pleasant, marvelous experience. Very often in the lesson, I say, "Look, would you stop? So many of you look so stern, as if you were trying to do something terrible, difficult, and unpleasant for you. That means you're tired, you won't understand any more. Break it, go and have a coffee, and stop it. Or let me tell you a story so that I can see the brightness in your eyes and a smile on your face, and that you'll listen and find that what I say is important to you."

WILL SCHUTZ: To me, that is very important, but it isn't the main thing you do. You do talk, and you do make these points, but the big thing is what goes on with the hands. To watch a Feldenkrais lesson for me is a meditation. It's very quiet and sensitive, and it's in the hands where the things happen. There's a communication from the body to the brain that's going on without any words, through the hands. The talk usually comes later.

In the process of working on the book, David Zemach-Bersin and I revisited the unedited version of the original New Dimensions interview. We found this story about Ben-Gurion[4] and Moshe Dayan[5] to be well worth including. Many thanks to Kaethe Zemach-Bersin for her editing work and to Jacqueline Rubinstein for the transcription.—Ed.

MOSHE FELDENKRAIS: It is a long story, but I can tell it as shortly as I can. Look, I worked with David Ben-Gurion; he learned with me. And he was taking lessons with me for about twenty years, the last twenty years of his life. And I believe that the changes in him were very profound. After he died, the foundation, the museum came to me and interviewed me, so that in the museum in the house where he lived, everyone who comes can press the button and listen to the story of how Ben-Gurion and I met and what happened and what I have to say about it. So when I worked with him, he always asked questions. He was a curious man. He was a man who learned all of his life. Ben-Gurion asked me one day to explain something. He said why do you do it that way? Why shouldn't you do it fast or strong like I do? So I explained to him. And he said, I don't really understand you quite clearly. . . .

At that time I didn't know Moshe Dayan. Because I was with Ben-Gurion, and Dayan was at that time the head of the army, the commander of the army, and he knew that I didn't know Dayan. So, I told him you know that I don't know him, but you know that he had a bullet that somebody shot through the binoculars into his eye in French Vichy Syria. He was in the Australian-British Army in Palestine. He was there fighting against the Vichy French. And someone shot him into that binocular and mutilated the eye. And how long is it since that happened? Fifteen years? I say, well, I can predict in another fifteen years, if he does not have it up till now, he will probably have headaches and his body will be distorted and he will have pain in the neck and he will have pain in the lower back. And, as he is a prominent and important person, he will go to the best surgeon in the hospital, and they will X-ray him and tell him that he needs a corset or they will do a traction and they will tell him that his spine is distorted.... And I tell you, even now, give me Dayan and I will make [it] that he will not have to be in the state that I have described. Because I will teach him something which he doesn't already know. And that was that. Ben-Gurion said all right. Dayan was at that time in Kenya or Africa, and he said when he is back, I will tell him. So I said, now you check it and you will see that I am right. And the most important thing is that this man will be treated as if he has spinal trouble, while his trouble is that his head and eyes are not properly aligned. And that will make all the trouble and nobody will be able to cure him. He will be treated as someone who has spondylosis or a scoliosis or some disc hernia. He will be treated like that. That could be prevented from the start. A few months later, I hear on the telephone, someone telephoned me, Ben-Gurion wants to talk to you. I didn't realize why he suddenly wants to talk to me. Maybe he wants to cancel, he can't come. He says, Moshe, I talked to Moshe and what you said would come in two years is already five years like that. And Moshe told me, that means Dayan told him, that he has such headaches and trouble that he has to drag himself to take painkillers to such a degree that till ten in the morning he doesn't know what people are saying to him. And so, you know what Ben-Gurion did? He told him, look, Dayan, you will go to Feldenkrais to have lessons with him. Dayan says, "I do not have time to do it. How can I come to Tel Aviv a different day? First, I want to go to the university in Jerusalem to study," which he did actually. So Ben-Gurion told him, "I am the Minister of Defense. This is an order. Moshe, you will go to Feldenkrais whether you want to or not. It is an order."

And then he came to me for many months, every time on a Friday coming from Jerusalem; he was at the university studying then. Now you want to know the thing he said—this is an intelligent man who loses an eye—what does he find? He finds that with one eye on one side he sees like before, but on the other side he knocks into things, doesn't see a telegraph post and doesn't see other things and knocks himself around. So obviously an intelligent man sees I haven't gotten an eye so I will tilt my head a little bit to the side, so my good eye can see symmetrically relative to the direction I am walking. Which is perfectly normal and correct. And all you had to do at the beginning would be to tell Dayan, look, you have lost your eye, to walk in the street, to drive you have to do that, but you must know if you persist like that you will destroy your entire body and you will have trouble in the back and pain and migraine and headaches; therefore, when you move, hold your head as you need to see properly, but you must know any second that you don't need it, you must regain the middle and your nose should guide you, not your good eye.

Therefore, if you do that intermittently, I can with two eyes look, turn the head and look to one side, if I drive on the right or on the left, I look one side, but that doesn't do any harm to anybody. The trouble is when you get a permanent deviation with no control. It means when it becomes a compulsive habit. Then of course your whole body fits itself to fit to the function of which you demand of it. Your brain, your muscles, your skeleton deforms to fulfill what your intentional cortex directs you to do.

Now, I needed to make him aware that actually his trouble depends on that. And that he can, even now, reverse the thing and relearn. Not relearn, learn something new. He can't recover the eye. He can't do it as he did before. He has to do it in a new way, but he can learn and do that. He is an intelligent, a super-intelligent man; how come he commits such a silly thing? And destroyed his own self completely. You see, there is nothing worse than ignorance. It is worse than being silly. Because when you are silly you don't know the difference between good and bad, but with ignorance you can intentionally do harm to yourself.

13

The Forebrain: Sleep, Consciousness, Awareness, and Learning

Interview with Edward Rosenfeld

Edward Rosenfeld is the author of *The Book of Highs: 250 Methods for Altering Your Consciousness Without Drugs*, so perhaps it's not surprising that awareness and consciousness are central themes in this interview. He was accompanied by two psychotherapists, Bennett L. Shapiro and Marty Fromm. The interview took place September 17, 1973.–*Ed.*

EDWARD ROSENFELD: We're talking with you for an article that will be in a magazine called *Consciousness,* and I understand that you've had a lot of words like "consciousness" thrown at you all day. We don't know what "consciousness" is; we are searching for a variety of approaches that might help define for us and for the people who read the magazine what "consciousness" is.

MOSHE FELDENKRAIS: That is actually a very nice, honest statement because I hear people talk and write about "consciousness"—whoever I asked what it is, they don't have the faintest idea—just a word—and with that word they go on to "old consciousness" and "new consciousness"—old thing I don't know what it is and new thing I don't know what it is. What does it mean?

I have always, in my own work, in everything I do—I say a word and say that's an unfolding process. How does a process unfold? We'll start simply. To me, human existence has four states and not others. These are sleeping, and the state of being awake, and the state of consciousness, and the state of awareness—and they are not the same. Now what's the difference between any of those? Roughly speaking, when we're asleep it means that what happens in the brain detaches itself from, first of all, time—from temporal function. Time is detached in such a way that it does not have its normal, serial, sequential order. It means something happens in the brain where it's not necessary that the next minute should follow the minute before. The next thing that's missing is orientation. The person detaches himself from orientation. I don't think about eyes detaching themselves from seeing and hearing, which helps to see. There are some people who sleep with open eyes, and some sleep through any noise, provided that the noise is not something of vital interest. (For instance, if a mother hears her child crying, no matter how deeply she sleeps, she will wake up.) That is sleep. For instance, you can't fly in reality, but in your sleep you can fly.

ER: What about people who talk in their sleep?

MF: If you want to complicate it, what about somnambulism? What about hypnotism? What about anything? If you want to complicate it, we'll never finish the interview!

ER: Okay, sorry.

MF: So, now we have sleep. Sleep means withdrawal. In sleep, time and space must be disrupted. If this is not happening the person is not asleep. And he won't dream, because in these dreams he must have time so distorted that what happened yesterday can be connected with childish memories, with feeling and sensations that he doesn't know, connected with excess acidity in the stomach, with tension in the back (if he lies on his back and warms his lower back, he may have an erection and dream about God knows what). It has nothing to do with reality. The withdrawal from life must be complete—it is desirable for better sleep. The withdrawal of the body from the sense of touch is more or less complete, but not entirely. If someone is asleep and you pour lukewarm water on his feet, he will micturate [urinate]. If you put something hard under his leg, he will change position even though he is asleep. When he wakes up he is not conscious; he has just woken up. If he has not picked up the time sequence, or, first of all, the orientation, he needs to find out where he is in relation to the vertical, relative to his standing position with the eyes horizontal. If this doesn't happen he is unable to move or know where he is. If a person sleeps and knows at the moment he falls asleep where objects are around him, and you change it while he is asleep, or if he changes position in bed, he wakes up and he cannot orient himself. He feels completely lost to the point of being afraid to move. He doesn't actually know what he experiences. Is this a table or is it something else? He doesn't know what it is.

Therefore, there is a state which is similar to sleep, the state I call "being awake." Before you have made contact, or realize how you are oriented to the room, you have no control over your body. This has no relation to consciousness. This means he knows the relation of space to himself—he knows where he is—where his right is and where his left is—where his up and down are. This is the lowest state of consciousness. Consciousness like this does not exist in animals—only in human beings. For what reason? Because the structure in humans is more complex. What structure is responsible for consciousness? It is the forebrain, which is asymmetrical and distinct from all other parts of the brain. The reticular system, the limbic system—they are all completely symmetrical. Their connections are also different, and their speed of functioning is different. They are all faster than the forebrain. All the others are symmetrical, fast, and connected very richly with the thalamus—that means with feelings, with moods, with attitudes. The reticular system has all the connections you can think of.

The limbic system is mostly serial. All the synapses, the axons, are always serial, one after another. Now, in the forebrain, most of the connections are in parallel and they are slow—about ten times slower than in all the other parts of the nervous system. They are asymmetrical. They have very poor integration with the thalamus. This asymmetry makes it possible to recognize the difference between right and left—opposition. And we have a tendency to divide everything into oppositions, which is idiotic and infantile.

For instance, we say light and dark as if light is the opposite of dark, which it isn't. Dark is the absence of light and not the opposite of light. You can see that the space outside, which has plenty of light from the sun, is still not lighted; it's dark. Cold and warm are not opposite. Cold is just a little less warm than warm, and that there is less mobility of atoms and electrons when it is cold. This is not an opposition. Korzybski[1] has already pointed out that this is infantile thinking. This comes from that structure of ours which demands simple opposition. From the beginning, when a child discovers this, he is very intrigued. A baby will turn and twist and taste for hours because something is different, and this is asymmetry which they can't resolve. We get used to it, but the mystery persists. How come you can't put a right hand into a left glove? It's idiotic but it's so. Mathematicians of genius have tried to solve it, and they say if you take a fourth dimension you can solve it, but if you say a fourth dimension it means nothing to anyone. All right, you have a forebrain, which is capable of functioning slower than the others, which is asymmetrical, which has direct control over parts because it is connected in parallel, it can override unconscious, primitive reactions. Being slower, it has the possibility, like every newly walled layer in the nervous system, to have an influence on the rear brain. It can modulate it for making more gradation, greater differentiation, slower understanding, finer perception. And that's what our consciousness does. Therefore, the forebrain is working slower, and can realize what is happening in the body and stop it or enhance it. For instance, now you make like that with the head, it is because you have seen, realized, and you wanted to say, "Yes." But you could have, you may want to smile now and inhibit it or enhance it. Stop yourself from smiling. That couldn't be if your thought was fast. You can see it in your normal life. When you walk and slip on something or walk on a step which isn't there, then your body reacts immediately, but you don't know what it is. It's only afterwards, with the slow brain that has observed what you have done and tells you that you are in a state I call "consciousness."

ER: I know when I have those kinds of experiences and when I step for a step that isn't there, it's almost like a shock.

MF: It is a shock.

ER: So you are saying that it's the forebrain that brings on that kind of shock?

MF: No, every superior layer in evolution, which means the one above the lowest (where Jackson has shown that it is actually above when the body stands) is not only later in time, but higher in structure. That's why the words "higher [nervous] centers" became familiar. But the forebrain does not work as fast as the old, primitive parts of the brain. They have fifty or sixty million years' experience, and through evolution, mutation, and survival of the fittest have worked up to be very strong, stable, reliable machinery. But the forebrain is a recent structure in the human brain. Consciousness is a new phenomenon in the brain—in nature in general—and therefore is weak. It gives better gradation, finer appreciation, greater variety. But for quick reaction we must depend on the old brain, because by the time you decide that's a banana peel and what to do with it, you will break your neck. Or if you are driving your car and you come to a patch of oil, by the time you decide it's a patch of oil you will long ago have been killed. This is primarily because of the asymmetry, the slowness. Another thing—we said it is very poorly integrated with the thalamus and this means it doesn't work where there are violent emotions. If you are angry, you have no conscious control over yourself and you think like an idiot. When the thalamus is irritated, the forebrain has very little chance of doing anything. The excitation diffuses and the higher, delicate control gives up. Then you find all sorts of tricks like counting or closing your eyes to reduce the excitation that is overrunning the forebrain. Thus you can regain conscious control over yourself; otherwise, you have no control.

But it shows you that clear thinking must be without emotion. When you are jealous, your thinking is mad. When you are afraid your thinking is worth nothing—you can't solve problems. When you are angry, jealous, afraid, when you have anxieties, your thinking is worse than the thinking of a dog when he runs away from a stick.

Now you can see that in that way consciousness becomes much more tangible, much more real than just a word, "consciousness." You can see that if the consciousness is poor, it has little awareness of the body. That is the whole thing. The quality of the consciousness is the ability to find what the other nervous centers do. Your hand is the same as any ape's, only you can't educate the ape to do fine-quality work like playing the violin or writing, or the work of a diamond cutter or polisher. This is a quality of work which needs certain powers of observation. And painting, drawing—it's the same thing. I take a piece of paper, I look at you, and what do I do? I weigh the hand—will the hand obey me to transcribe what I see or not? Then it is reduced in size so that the movement is topologically correct but the scale is not correct. Then I must observe myself, feel whether my hand is doing what I am seeing—and judge relationships. Where is your eyebrow in relation to your hair? How far is it from the mouth? That is consciousness. You must observe yourself and relate your sensations. The moving of your outer attention inward—through the eyes and ears and touch—that is "consciousness."

MARTY FROMM: What is awareness then? How does that come into it?

MF: Awareness is that part of the consciousness which involves knowledge. For instance, we are all sitting here. Can you tell me if you are sitting at an equal distance from her or from him? You know it—you see it, but you don't know. When will you know? When you observe what you judge with the movement of your eyes. That's knowledge. Before, you had a faint idea— that's consciousness. But you don't know whether they are equal or not. You don't know in many other respects. For instance, you don't know how many doors there are in this room. You saw them. How many steps there are in your house—you walked them a million times. How many windows are there in the house you live in? In the house you were born in? How many tiles? You don't know—you don't need it. But if you needed to know what would you do? You will go and count them. How will you count them? You will observe how many acts of change there are, movements of the eyes, or movement of the finger, or actual movement of the head, or movement of the attention. And you can even do it in your imagination. In your imagination you can present it and say, "Look—there's the first door and there's the door on the right . . . ," and what you are doing is scanning what your consciousness knows it has done a million times, but you can't bring it into an orderly knowledge unless you are aware.

The moments of awareness are normally very rare for most people. Those people who have produced, created, transformed the world in which we live have improved their awareness. For instance, some people have found out that this pencil is actually made out of porous material—out of atoms. And it took them a good many years to see that atoms are the smallest matter that can divide. In 1943 I predicted something that all the world knows now; something that all scientists say now; that was said before anyone knew there was a hydrogen bomb. I said at that time that there is a nucleus and protons and atoms. [Moshe Feldenkrais made this observation in his first book, *Body and Mature Behavior.*]

BENNETT L. SHAPIRO: The Rutherford–Bohr atom.

MF: Yes, and I said in the book that they were all a band of idiots, the scientists, because what they studied—the particles—have such a short life, and now we know.... When I look at the things I knew at that time I can't understand how I did.

BLS: You presented this material for the first time in 1943.

MF: It was something which nobody was interested in.

BLS: What impressed me, having read that book very carefully, was that there are still some things in it that people aren't aware of. I particularly like this thing you said on page 32. You said, "... Life, as well as the material world, will probably never be reduced to something very simple unless an entirely new method of thinking, not based on causality, is developed ..."

MF: Today everybody knows it. There are many things here that I was twenty-five years ahead of [my] time with. That is why I am such a misery, in that I become known when I am going to die already. Anyway, you will see here that it is written that it is idiotic to think there are only electrons, protons, and neutrons, and if we look closer we can see that there are thousands of particles which form and die and that there are such a variety—we know only those which are very stable.

I think it's possible to improve consciousness because "consciousness," as I define it, is the quality of observing by the higher nervous center what is happening in the lower ones. And this, observing, was done to only the useful things that humanity found essential to the long, miserable life that it has had up till now. Up till the last few decades, people had no time to deal with consciousness—they dealt only with immediate appetites: eat, see, and grab—and that's why consciousness was only in the fingers, in the mouth and eyes, and a little bit in the genitals. It was a great work by Freud that he discovered trouble in those parts—he called it anal state and oral state and that's a man who did it only in words—in thinking and feeling. When he speaks about unconsciousness he says the same things that I tell you about consciousness—that it's anal, oral, genital—that's all—and manipulative, which he left out because he didn't think properly. He didn't understand the proper problem. And in his way of trying to solve the problem, he introduced schizophrenia in everybody—the id, ego, and superego. You have three personalities. Now who are you?

ER: Does the fact that the forebrain allows us that moment of pause, that fine tuning, make available a unified consciousness—rather than a split consciousness? Rather than lots of different oral, anal, genital fragments?

MF: It can be, but our culture has never recognized it—it has trained the human being as if he were one of those primitive structures, like an animal, like a dog, like a machine, and in better states like a telephone—like the behaviorists want him to be, only action-reaction. But ask the behaviorists one question—how come a rat, a mouse, a kitten, and a human being are born with curiosity? Why do they look about after they have eaten everything? What pushes a human being to know? Curiosity is something that goes from the inside out, not the other way around—and it exists before you have experience. It exists in a baby, before he can do anything. It exists in all animals. That is the first law in that machine-telephone exchange—

that something impinges on you, you have a stimulus and you are conditioned and you have a response. Conditioned reflexes work only when there is satisfaction to the stimulus. If you give a dog the meat and then ring the bell, he won't respond again. If you ring the bell and then give him the meat within three seconds you will teach him to salivate at the bell. This condition doesn't exist in human beings who have imagination. If you give the dog the food and then ring the bell, you will never form a conditioned reflex. In human beings, once you do it, he can think and change the order. If he changes the order it is ineffective.

FROMM: Who were your teachers?

MF: Myself. I refused to go to the university to learn medicine. I refused to be wired-in like everybody else. I said I don't mind making my own mistakes, but I don't want to learn by the authority of a known professor. He will convince me because he knows better and in half a year I will lose all my curiosity. I'll be learning like everybody else—and get a good diploma.

ER: When were you born?

MF: In 1904, the sixth of May.

ER: Where?

MF: Where? In a bed.

ER: What city or town, what country?

MF: I changed nationalities three times before I was thirteen. First it was Polish, then German, then Russian. Now I think it is something between the last two.

ER: How old were you when you went to Israel?

MF: I went to Israel in 1918, when I was fourteen. I went by myself—all alone.

ER: And you said it took twelve years of work previous to these lectures before *Body and Mature Behavior* was done. [This is Dr. Feldenkrais's first published book about his *Method.—Ed.*]

MF: I worked on myself, healing my own knees. They were troubling me and the doctors said that the operation would make them stiff.

ER: So it was your own physical disability which prompted you to learn?

MF: Yes. I thought I would read up on the structure and in that way I would solve the problem myself.

ER: When did you move out of doing physics full-time into bodywork?

MF: Never. I never moved out. There was a period of about seven years when I gave up this and went back to physics . . . then I went to Israel and worked in the science army of the Israeli Defense Forces, and I formed the Electronics Department of the force. They brought me there for that purpose.

ER: Have you been training people to be able to do the kind of individual work that you do?

MF: Yes. I formed one group. It had fourteen people. The first group I trained took three years—daily—two hours with me and two hours under my supervision. They were working on each other and on me. Trying out on me the techniques even if they couldn't do them properly. We work in order to increase the sensitivity of our hands and the awareness that can be read when our hands touch the body. We are looking for minor differences— degenerate tissues, muscles that are permanently protracted, infiltration in the fascia. This needs not only delicacy, but knowing what you touch. Any person, if he is told to touch ten hands in one particular way, will know that they are all different. He has the sensitivity but he hasn't got the skill of mine to know what he is doing. To teach him what he is feeling I have to improve his own self-knowledge. Therefore, I have to work with everyone with my hands, each one separately, coaching them and at the same time increasing their self-awareness and their skill of appreciation.

ER: Are you trying to compress the training period down to one year?

MF: I am not trying to compress. The thing is this—in the first group there were some people who learned with extraordinary ease. One of them was a professor of inorganic chemistry; another was a neurologist and psychiatrist and is the head of a mental hospital. But there were others who needed time to learn. All of the people, after we had finished and after they had done individual work for up to one year, asked to have an additional month together because they realized things that they didn't appreciate before and because they found new things that they wanted to test. It is the same with a young doctor who gets out of medical school and practices medicine, but still sends people to the hospital because there are things that he doesn't rely on himself for.

ER: How long is your training period now?

MF: I haven't done any training recently.

ER: Are you starting another group?

MF: I should, but I have very great difficulties here in America. People here think that they can "marathon" everything. Marathon workshops, marathon learning—two weeks at a time. Some of them are learning in two weeks and then teaching.

14

An Interview with Moshe Feldenkrais

The New Sun

The New Sun was a monthly publication concerned with spirituality, health, and alternative lifestyles. Founded in 1976, it was one of the first of its kind in the United States. The interview was conducted in New York in 1977 by *The New Sun* staff: Bruce Silvey, Eliot Sobel, and Chana Benjamin.—*Ed.*

Before the interview began, we were privileged to watch Feldenkrais working on a client—a woman who, we learned, was suffering from an advanced cancer. She appeared to be very elated and grateful at the end of her brief session.

THE NEW SUN: Did her change of mood come about through your work on her body?

MOSHE FELDENKRAIS: I don't work on the body. I work on the person, not on the body. I don't know a body without a person.

NS: It appeared to be that you were working with bones, with the spine, with muscles ...

MF: No, no, how can you work on a bone? What do you do to a bone? I work on the person, which means to reorganize his mood, his understanding ... look, I've never seen a person who didn't think, feel, sense, and move as one action—I never met one where those things were separate. You separate them in speaking and in writing, but now, you are here—are you here with your body or with your brain?

NS: All together.

MF: ... Therefore, how can you tell me ... look, I'll give you an idiotic example: if I amputate your body of one leg, who's the cripple?

NS: The leg or the body?

MF: Or you! I'm dealing with you, not with the leg and not with the muscles, and not with the nervous system, but with the overall person, and with the feeling and understanding and your image of yourself, and everything else.

NS: Okay, from a physiological standpoint, what is it that your hands are doing to that person?

MF: Making her aware of thinking, and feeling, and sensing, and body.

NS: Is it different for everyone?

MF: Of course.

NS: How do you know where to go on each person?

MF: When you will have my experience and knowledge you will also know.

NS: Obviously it comes from your experience and years of work with this.

MF: No, it comes from the theory, first of all. Many people work with bodies; why don't they do the same thing? Nobody does what I do. Obviously it doesn't come from working with people. When you have a theory, then your experience teaches and qualifies your understanding and your future experience. That's how science works.

NS: Let's look at it from the standpoint of readers who are going to be reading an interview with you and . . . Please explain your work to us. . . .

MF: I consider a human being to be pieces of bone that never had any say about how to align themselves any more than bricks know how to build a house. So bones can't do it. Muscles can only contract and stop contracting. If muscles contracted, all of them together, what sort of human being would you have? He couldn't sit or do anything. Just contract and de-contract. So what? Therefore, you need a brain; you need a nervous system that will distribute the impulses so as to contract the body in one way or another—standing, sitting, walking, doing whatever a person may do. But the brain itself, can it speak? Can you walk? Can you write? Can you whis-tle? Can you sing? Can you make music? When a human being is born, out-side of the physiological functions he was born with to survive, like breathing, there is nothing. I repeat, he can't write, he can't speak, he can't make music, he doesn't know what time it is. But the brain will learn; you learned English—how?

NS: I was taught it.

MF.: You weren't taught it; nobody taught you English in the beginning.

NS: I heard.

MF: You heard. Did you? But how did you learn?

NS: Repetition.

MF: Nobody repeated the same thing to you.

NS: Well, I heard, for example, my own name, being called that constantly.

MF: And how long did it take before you realized that you are not a name? All right, then, you speak English because you heard English. Your nervous system was wired-in to English early through your own experience in childhood. All of the other things were wired-in through the experience of that nervous system in the environment. Therefore, the real important thing is the environment, the nervous system, the muscles, and the bones. The real important thing is the wiring-in, the learning process. All I've done is seen clearly that in that complete loop, you cannot neglect anything if you want to make any improvement in that being.

NS: So if I have a problem it's probably a break in the link somewhere.

MF: Why a break? As the whole thing is learned, it is learned from people who didn't teach you—it just happened, it's chance, your luck, you have no say in it. Therefore it can be good, it can be bad. And if nobody's aware of the process, either, then everybody grows up and believes that that's the way it is. He's got ideas inherited from the surroundings—that the body is something else and the mind is something else and the skeleton is something else—and you devise a million different systems, each one dealing with a particular thing which is of no consequence.

NS: Do you think we are totally victims of fate?

MF: Why victims? We are the authors! You are also the victim and the doer. Because some people have stopped and thought. Leonardo da Vinci stopped and thought, Freud stopped and thought, Zarathustra stopped and thought. But some don't. So they remain . . .

NS: Machines.

MF: Machine-like. Intelligent machines, very clever machines, IBM first-rate computers. But they still need somebody to put in them a kind of ticket, or punched card, and they function with that. I believe a human being has free choice, and he can't have free choice unless he has alternative ways of doing the same thing. If he has no alternative ways, then what's his free choice?

NS: Did you come to a point in your life when you noticed that you were machine-like and you did something about it?

MF: Oh, yes, from early childhood I knew I was a machine. I saw other people being completely machine-like.

NS: And what did you do about it?

MF: I didn't know what to do. I did what you do—try to find out, and found out it didn't work, so I became a scientist like everyone else.

NS: Generally speaking, a person does not know what to do about that. If he comes to you he can find out some of the possibilities. If he can't get to you ...

MF: It's neither as simple nor complex as that. In fact, I don't know a person who does not find fault with himself. I don't know a person who doesn't find fault with his eyesight, and I don't know a person who doesn't find fault with his posture, I don't know a person who doesn't find fault with his breathing, and I don't know a person who thinks that his life is as good as he can make it and as he would wish it. Therefore, everybody feels that he's fucked somewhere, and really has no choice. So what does he do? He keeps on doing the same thing; he has no choice. But the people who come to me come not knowing what I am going to teach them. None of them. They come when their trouble becomes so great that they feel they need help, so they go and look for it. So they go to Bioenergetics, they go to analysis, they go to meditation, they go to fifty systems and they do all of them together— they do tai chi and they do aikido, and they go swimming, and meditation and yoga, everything. And then they hear that somebody is teaching something which is neither this, nor that, nor that, and they feel very funny about it. So those who seek—and most of the people who do all these things are actually the people who know very well that they have not realized their potential, they have not made their life and themselves a harmonious whole— those come to me. And they come to me usually because they have some trouble which is beyond repair by every other system. And I teach them what I think is the most important thing, to make them into human beings who have a free will and a free choice. That means everything that they know how to do, I teach them another way of doing.

NS: Now you say you work on the person . . .

MF: I work *with* the person.

NS: With the person. What we saw was movement of the body.

MF: No, that is your mistake. How could I work with the body! The person came to me . . .

NS: You don't make a separation between . . .

MF: How could I? If I could have the body alone I could take it in a coffin and take it with me. And if I did to that body anything without the brain . . . cut off the head, you'll see that whatever I did was worth nothing.

NS: That form of working with a person seems to change their emotions and their viewpoint.

MF: How could it be otherwise? Right now, that you are listening to me, does it change your attention, your understanding, your feeling, sensing, and sitting, and movement? And look at your hand! I can see in your fingers the way and what you think now. Is it your body that makes that gesture? Or is it your state of mind and the mood and the way you think and your curiosity—that's what folds your hand like that. . . .

NS: When I put myself in a posture of attention like this, partly the posture helps me be more attentive, and partly it's a reflection of the fact that I'm paying attention.

MF: But you are wired-in like that. That can be changed. That's your posture of attention. It doesn't mean that it's the best for you now, but that's the one you know; you don't know another one, you have no choice, and therefore you are machine-like.

NS: I understand that you and Jean Houston* are going to work on a book together?

MF: We have already done so. It's called *Jean Houston Interviews Feldenkrais on Learning.* It's about the process of learning, what I understand by learning—not academic learning; it has nothing to do with academic learning.

NS: Can a person take that information and perhaps relearn some of the things?

MF: You can relearn all the time. You have learned a lot yourself. You have changed a lot since your parents brought you to school. You have made a lot of your own decisions and you have learned in the way which made the person you are now.

NS: What could a person do to change that?

MF: He need not change. It's not a question of changing. It's a question of becoming, knowing himself, and using himself in such a way that he does not regret the past few years for what he hasn't done, or the future for that matter. It means he feels the way a tree in a field feels—it's part of nature. The tree by itself would not live, the earth without trees could not live, and a human being should feel the same way—that he's part of this world.

---

*Dr. Jean Houston co-directed the Foundation for Mind Research with her husband Dr. Robert Masters. They were leaders in the human potential movement and early supporters of Feldenkrais.

NS: If I came here and I was depressed, and I looked gloomy, what would you do?

MF: I would ask, are you sad all the time?

NS: No.

MF: No, then how did you know when you fixed the appointment three days ago that you would be sad when you came in? You see, we take words for things, and once we got them as a thing, we find that the thing doesn't work as we wish. Because a word means a million different things to every other person. You say sad and you want me to treat sadness. I can't treat sadness. Sadness is an expression of something—your sadness and my sadness and his sadness are three different things. Everybody's sadness is a different thing. I will never be sad for the same thing as you. Therefore, when you say sadness, I can't do anything to sadness. But, a person being sad, I can do something to the person: how does he behave to bring about sadness?

NS: But isn't there a difference when you're working with, let's say, old age and with the whole group of problems associated with old age: rheumatism, arthritis . . .

MF: No, you're mistaken. When you say that, you again make words into things, as if arthritis and old age go together.

NS: So instead of saying, "I have arthritis; what can you do about it?" you would say, "Arthritis I don't know about; you, I can work with."

MF: Yes, I can make you tick in such a way that you don't have arthritis.

NS: When you start to work with someone, what are your clues to tell you where they're at?

MF: I have in my mind, through my theory, worked out the system I told you about. We have an environment and a nervous system and muscles and bones, and the nervous system growing in the environment has curiosity and tries to cope with what happens around it, being touched, being given a name, hearing words; it has to pee and breathe and ... All that together will gradually work itself into a complete closed loop, so a person without an environment cannot live. The environment without a person means nothing, means the interstellar cosmos—the bones without the muscles means nothing, the muscles without the nervous system means nothing, the muscles and the nervous system without the environment means nothing.

Now you can imagine what happens now: each being like that is by chance or luck or astrological determination born at a given time, and the only thing that makes some order in this world of chaos, of chance, of no say at all, is a nervous system. It makes cause and effect in some things; it finds a continuity and builds a system that works and can maintain itself for sixty or seventy or eighty years.

The idea, therefore, when you ask me what do I do when I work with a person, is this: through long thinking, and touching, and feeling, and sensing, and working, and moving with other people, I found out that it is possible to imagine a theoretical, nonexistent system—a system where each bone is as perfect as can be in anatomical perfection. The muscles are the best the world has ever seen (which do not exist) and they are connected in the most beautiful way to those bones. Then there's the nervous system, which has the greatest ability, greatest facility for wiring itself in to any kind of thing that you want—because you know there are about three thousand different professions in the human species, and two thousand languages—and I imagine an ideal environment. Not like your father and your mother or my father and my mother to whom every analyst will find that all my inhibitions and all my complexes are due, and therefore you find to my mind the idiotic state where everybody who has a father and mother must be analyzed until they find out what's wrong with that [damn] father and mother. A human being must have parents, and must live with them and must like them and must hate them and must honor them and despise them, and everything else. But he must be capable of rendering his own life interesting, full, rich, and satisfying to himself.

So, I have an ideal environment, which is again nonexistent, and I imagine: what would a human being be like who had an ideal structure, ideal environment, and ideal learning process? Now when I am with a person, I look, hear, listen, know. I can see the structure, I can see the way he addresses himself to me, I can hear what he says—you wouldn't believe how informative a person's approach is. With that I can find the first outstanding deviation from the ideal being that I described to you. Therefore, I take that gross error and make him aware of it—sometimes with my hands, sometimes with an observation. I use everything I have: my eyes, my ears, my hands, my mouth. Once you've eliminated one of those gross errors, you find that a person is already astonished: How did you find out that that bothers me? And it is the most outstanding, most difficult thing that that person carries with him without being aware of it. He talks about anything else except that. For instance, somebody phoned and said, "For two years I've had a headache." But surely, *headache* is a word. Headache means too much blood comes to the brain and to the scalp, and she brings that about. How? She hasn't got the faintest idea. I don't know what to do with a headache. Each human being has a headache for a different reason and in a different way. When you bring to me the environment, the nervous system, thinking, speaking, feeling, sensing, and moving, in any one of them I can find the gross deviation from that ideal thing, and that I will make them aware of.

NS: Do you start out by seeing a person and imagining who they would be if they lived in the ideal world?

MF: Yes, but if I stopped like that to figure it out I would never be able to do anything. That is already in my system. It took me fifteen years to work out the ideal system, so I know it inside out. You don't believe that I could work out a system like that without having to change my entire understanding of who I am and what I am doing and how I think and how I move—finding out, actually, that I was wired-in, that I had no say in what I was doing. Once I discovered that, I found that every word I said didn't really mean what I said. And actually, I could find out what you say now, you don't really mean.

212

You said sad and then two minutes later you saw it was nonsense. It is our common condition that concerns all human beings—that's why it also interests me. Not because I have something to make you feel better or me feel better. In fact, I don't have sympathy for the people I work with who come to me in such dreadful states. My only feeling is this: we, the person and I, have a common enemy: ignorance and chance, over which we have no say. Against that we have only one extraordinary means: the human nervous system, which is capable, in conjunction with other nervous systems, to form a kind of order which enables us to live in a hostile world.

NS: If everybody has a headache for a different reason, does that mean you cannot give a general prescription?

MF: Woooo, you want a general prescription, go to a doctor. To him you can say I have a headache and he'll give you aspirin.

NS: So you couldn't say that something which usually works for a headache is to do this or that?

MF: Ohhhh, nothing at all, never. All those people go to fifty doctors and get aspirin and Anacin with twenty-three percent more headache-fighting ... all that ... they don't come to me so long as anybody can help them. To me they come when they've exhausted the whole thing and it doesn't work. And then they come to me and I don't do anything against the headache, because the headache is nothing. What is a headache? How can you do something with a headache? What can you do to it? Take it away? Show me a headache that you took out! You cured it? Where is it? What did you do to the headache? I am only a human being. I can deal with a human being who tells me that he feels some trouble in his head, which is a different thing than a headache being cured. Therefore, the answer is nowhere, nowhere, at no time, have I had a specific treatment for anything.

NS: What we've been talking about partly is your general approach to a person who comes in and says, "Help me."

MF: No, for then I say, "What can I do for you?"

NS: All right, then they tell you, but how do you know what to do?

MF: How do you know how to swallow? Tell me how you swallow, then I will tell you how I know. Answer me.

NS: It comes naturally.

MF: Then to me it comes naturally to think and be clever. To me it comes naturally to understand, feel, sense, and do.

NS: Thank you, Dr. Feldenkrais.

Notes

Chapter 1

1. Michael Wolgensinger has published more than twenty acclaimed books on photography, with *Zurich* and *Spain* being two of the better-known titles. Feldenkrais often stayed at the Wolfensingers' home for weeks at a time and treated it like a second home when he was in Europe. During these visits Wolgensinger took many photographs and we are grateful to his daughter Lea Wolgensinger for her permission to include her father's photos in this collection.

2. George Ivanovich Gurdjieff (1866–1949) was an Armenian-Greek spiritual teacher who taught in the early part of the twentieth century mainly in Russia and France. Feldenkrais was quite interested in his approach and had extensive interactions with many of his disciples. Gurdjieff taught that most people spend their lives in a waking sleep and that special efforts of attention and self-observation were needed to awaken. The "Stop" exercise referred to here by Feldenkrais was one of many practices working to that end. In addition, "The Work" (as Gurdjieff's approach was referred to) utilizes a sophisticated form of movement work combined with awareness practices, meditation, and intensive community interaction to cultivate inner development. Gurdjieff taught that there were three centers—thinking, feeling, and moving—and an important goal of The Work is forging a balance between them.

Chapter 2

1. For details about Gurdjieff, see note 2 above. Peter Ouspensky (1878–1947) was one of Gurdjieff's original followers, who separated himself from Gurdjieff and formed his own group. He is best known for authoring *In Search of the Miraculous,* an account of his first exposure to Gurdjieff and what he learned in his ten years studying with him.

Chapter 4

1. Feldenkrais received his DSc degree from the Sorbonne University in Paris, where he met Frédéric Joliot-Curie. Frédéric was married to Irène Curie,

the daughter of the famous scientist Marie Curie, and they took the combined last name of Joliot-Curie. The husband and wife Joliot-Curie team received a Nobel Prize in Chemistry in 1935 for their work on the structure of the atom. Feldenkrais worked with them in their lab during the 1930s.

Chapter 5

1. Heinz von Foerster (1911–2002) was an Austrian-American scientist whose work, Feldenkrais found, intersected with his own. Dr. von Foerster is known as one of the architects of cybernetics and as an important contributor to the theories of systemics and constructivism. Constructivism is an educational theory stressing the importance of the student's personal construction of knowledge through problem solving and direct experience. Dr. von Foerster was invited to present in Feldenkrais's San Francisco training program in 1977 and he gave a keynote address at one of the Feldenkrais Guild conferences. He has had many fruitful exchanges with the Feldenkrais community, including this editor, who remembers him very fondly.

2. Henri Poincaré (1854–1912) was a mathematician, physicist, and philosopher of science with a particular interest in phenomenology. He was enormously productive and creative and has had a lasting impact in many of the areas in which he worked. Among his many interests was a curiosity about perception leading to the work Feldenkrais refers to here.

3. Wolfgang Köhler (1887–1967) was a German psychologist and one of the founders of Gestalt psychology. He is well known for his experiments with inversion goggles referred to here by Feldenkrais.

Chapter 6

1. Igor Markevitch (1912–1983) was an accomplished composer and conductor. He created more than twenty-five original compositions, being rated among the leading contemporary European composers in the 1930s. In the 1940s he devoted himself exclusively to conducting, working with many of Europe's major orchestras.

2. Peter Brook (1925–) is one of the most respected theater directors in Europe today, having had a long, varied, and innovative career. Brook's

work was influenced by the ideas of G. I. Gurdjieff and it may have been in this context that he met Feldenkrais. They had a long acquaintance and Brook had Feldenkrais teach his theater group annually for many years.

Chapter 7

1. Field Marshal Jan Christiaan Smuts (1870–1950) was a prominent statesman, military leader, and philosopher. He is also referred to as a genius maverick! He was the prime minister of South Africa, fought in both world wars as a field marshal, and was the visionary behind the League of Nations, for which he wrote the Preamble. He was also one of the architects of the United Nations. Here Moshe is referring to Smuts' 1926 book *Holism and Evolution,* where he coins the term *holism,* which he defines as "the tendency in nature to form wholes that are greater than the sum of the parts through creative evolution."

2. Milton Trager, MD (1908–1997) was the developer of the Trager® somatic system, which has philosophical overlaps with Feldenkrais's approach. Dr. Trager was present at the Mandala Conference where Feldenkrais delivered this talk. This was the first time they had met, and they exchanged hands-on sessions. In the comment referenced here Feldenkrais is referring to the fact that Dr. Trager received his MD in his late forties.

3. Johann Carl Gauss (1777–1855) was a scientist and mathematician, considered one of the best mathematicians of all time. Pierre-Simon, Marquis de Laplace (1749–1827) was a mathematician and important contributor in the study of astronomy. Thomas Edison (1847–1931) was a prolific American inventor.

4. Frédéric Joliot-Curie (1900–1958) was a Nobel-Prize-winning physicist whom Feldenkrais worked with in Paris during the 1930s. See chapter 4 note for more information.

Chapter 11

1. G. I. Gurdjieff (1866–1949) was a Russian teacher who moved to the West with a number of disciples after the Russian Revolution. His intent was to bring his students from the "sleep" of their ordinary conscious state to an awake condition in which through the act of "self-remembering" they could act with self-knowledge. *See also note for chapter 1 on page 215.—Ed.*

2. P. W. Bridgman, *The Logic of Modern Physics,* New York: Macmillan Co., 1927.

3. In Einstein's theory of relativity there is no absolute time because to compare clocks or distances requires sending signals which move at a fixed speed. If clocks on one system are to be compared with another, the speed of one system relative to the other system, one would find the clocks on one system are slowed relative to the other in proportion to how close the speed of one system relative to the other is to the speed of the signals (speed of light).

4. In terms of the internal connections of the nervous system all the sensory surfaces send signals to the central nervous system and at the same time receive signals in return. In this there is no distinction between external and internal sensing parts and at the same time the cells of the sensory surfaces are not distinguishable from any other cells of the system in that they are part of internal loops.

5. I believe that what Katzir means here is that in development the child needs stability and constancy. Only after the establishment of a stable sense of self is it possible to consider alternative ways of perceiving and conceptualizing.

6. Katzir is here referring to the Heisenberg uncertainty principle, which states that measurements at the level of the very small (the atomic level) are interlocked so that measuring a position with great accuracy results in a lowering of accuracy in the measurement of momentum, and vice versa.

7. The point of view that only a small part of the brain is used by an adult human is no longer held by most neuroscientists today.

8. At the time of the discussion, it was still believed that conditioning was the best model for explaining basic human and animal learning. Today we might better describe fixed learned patterns as strong "attractors" in the language of dynamics.

9. In the 1930s American psychologist E. R. Guthrie developed the contiguity theory of learning based on association rather than on the conditioned reflex of Pavlov.

10. Guthrie's idea was that simple learning could take place with a single experience. If this was repeated with consistency, the learned action or movement would become a habit. Complex learning such as a skill involves a group of habits that achieve a result in many different and varied conditions. Thus learning was not simple repetition. ("Edwin R. Guthrie," Chapter 3 in W. S. Sahakian, *Psychology of Learning*, Chicago: Markham Pub. Co., 1970.)

11. Servo-mechanism: A more complex feedback system whose variables affect one another. It involves internal control as well as external control.

12. "Schema," as used by Piaget, refers to some form of cognitive structure. It could be an action pattern or a perception or a concept. The term is not used very much today, but in dynamic terms it can be designated as an "attractor pattern."

Chapter 12

1. Feldenkrais visited The Rusk Institute of Rehabilitation Medicine at New York University in 1969 to demonstrate his work. The Esalen trip was the first time he taught an extended experiential course in the United States.

2. Oscar Ichazo (1931–) is the Bolivian-born founder of the Arica School, which aims to help people overcome their identification with their own mechanistic thought and behavior patterns. Arica was part of the cultural zeitgeist at the time of this interview.

3. Yehudi Menuhin (1916–1999) was a conductor and violinist. He is commonly considered one of the twentieth century's greatest violin virtuosos. He took lessons from Feldenkrais over a period of many years and was a great supporter. Vladimir Horowitz (1903–1989) is considered one of the great piano players of the last century.

4. David Ben-Gurion (1886–1973) was one of the founding fathers of the State of Israel and its first Prime Minister, serving between 1948 and 1963, with the exception of 1954–1955. Feldenkrais worked with Ben-Gurion for many years and taught him to stand on his head. An election campaign publicity photograph of Ben-Gurion standing on his head on a Tel Aviv beach was seen worldwide. In Israel it was said that "Feldenkrais put Ben-Gurion on his head and Ben-Gurion put Israel on its feet."

5. Moshe Dayan (1915–1981) was a well-known military leader and politician in the early decades of Israel's existence, serving as Defense Minister and later as Foreign Minister. He wore an eye patch due to the injury that Feldenkrais describes here.

Chapter 13

1. Alfred Korzybski (1879–1950) was a Polish-American philosopher and scientist. He is best known for creating the system of general semantics,

which investigates human meaning-making by probing the act of abstracting and the use of semantic symbols. A famous Korzybski quote is "The map is not the territory; the word is not the thing defined."

Photographs

A Biography of Moshe Feldenkrais

By Mark Reese

Moshe Pinchas Feldenkrais was born on May 6, 1904, in Slavuta, in present-day Ukraine. When he was a small boy his family moved to the nearby town of Korets. By 1912 his family moved to Baranovich, in what is today Belarus. While Baranovich endured many World War I battles, Feldenkrais received his Bar Mitzvah, completed two years of high school, and received an education in the Hebrew language and Zionist philosophy. At the age of fourteen in 1918, Feldenkrais left by himself on a six-month journey to Palestine.

After arriving in 1919, Feldenkrais worked as a laborer until 1923, when he returned to high school to earn a diploma. While attending school he made a living by tutoring. After graduating in 1925, he worked for the British survey office as a cartographer. Feldenkrais was involved in Jewish self-defense groups, and after learning jujitsu he devised his own self-defense techniques. He hurt his left knee in a soccer match in 1929. While convalescing he wrote *Autosuggestion* (1930), a translation from English to Hebrew of C. Harry Brooks's work on Émile Coué's system of autosuggestion, together with two chapters that he wrote himself. He next published *Jujitsu* (1931), a book on self-defense.

In 1930 Feldenkrais went to Paris and enrolled in an engineering college, the Ecole des Travaux Publics des Paris. He graduated in 1933 with specialties in mechanical and electrical engineering. In 1933, after meeting Jigoro Kano, judo's founder, Feldenkrais began teaching jujitsu again, and started his training in judo. In 1933 he began working as a research assistant under Frédéric Joliot-Curie at the Radium Institute while studying for his Ingénieur-Docteur degree at the Sorbonne. From 1935 to 1937 he worked at the Arcueil-Cachan laboratories building a Van de Graaff generator, which was used for atomic fission experiments. In 1935 he published a revised, French edition of his Hebrew jujitsu book called *La défense du faible contre l'agresseur,* and in 1938 he published *ABC du Judo.* He received his judo black belt in 1936, and second degree rank in 1938. Feldenkrais married Yona Rubenstein in 1938. From 1939 to 1940 he worked under Paul Langevin doing research on magnetics and ultrasound.

Feldenkrais escaped to England in 1940, just as the Germans arrived in Paris. As a scientific officer in the British Admiralty, he conducted anti-submarine research in Scotland from 1940 to 1945. While there he taught judo and self-defense classes. In 1942 he published a self-defense manual, *Practical Unarmed Combat,* and *Judo.* Feldenkrais began working with himself to deal with knee troubles that had recurred during his escape from France, and while walking on submarine decks. Feldenkrais gave a series of lectures about his new ideas, began to teach experimental classes, and worked privately with some colleagues.

In 1946 Feldenkrais left the Admiralty, moved to London, and worked as an inventor and consultant in private industry. He took judo classes at the London Budokwai, sat on the International Judo Committee, and scientifically analyzed judo principles. He published his first book on his method, *Body and Mature Behavior,* in 1949, and his last book on judo, *Higher Judo,* in 1952. During his London period he studied the work of George Gurdjieff, F. M. Alexander, and William Bates, and went to Switzerland to study with Heinrich Jacoby.

Feldenkrais returned to Israel to direct the Israeli Army Department of Electronics from 1951 to 1953. Around 1954 he moved permanently to Tel Aviv and, for the first time, made his living solely by teaching his Method. He worked sporadically on the manuscript of *The Potent Self,* which he had begun in London. Around 1955 he permanently located his *Awareness Through Movement* classes in a studio on Alexander Yanai Street. He gave *Functional Integration* lessons in the apartment where his mother and brother lived. In early 1957 Feldenkrais began giving lessons to Israeli Prime Minister David Ben-Gurion.

In the late 1950s Feldenkrais presented his work in Europe and the United States. In the mid-1960s he published "Mind and Body" and "Bodily Expression." In 1967, he published *Improving the Ability to Perform* (titled *Awareness Through Movement* in its 1972 English-language edition). In 1968, near his family's apartment, he made a studio at 49 Nachmani Street as the permanent site for his *Functional Integration* practice, and the location for his first teacher-training program, 1969–1971, given to twelve students.

After giving month-long courses internationally, he taught a sixty-five-student teacher-training program in San Francisco over four summers, 1975–1978. He published *The Case of Nora* in 1977, and *The Elusive Obvious* in 1981. He began the 235-student Amherst training in 1980 but was only able to teach the first two summers of the four-year program. After becoming ill in the fall of 1981, he stopped teaching publicly. He died on July 1, 1984.

I have done my best to verify dates, names, and places, though I cannot guarantee their accuracy, due to limitations of information available and discrepancies between sources.

—MR

Mark Reese has extensively researched Feldenkrais's life and is the author of an upcoming biography of Feldenkrais: *Moshe Feldenkrais: A Life in Movement.—Ed.*

About Elizabeth Beringer

Elizabeth Beringer has been involved with the practice and development of the *Feldenkrais Method* for more than thirty years. She studied directly with the founder of the Method, Dr. Moshe Feldenkrais, in both the United States and in Israel between 1976 and 1983. Over the years Elizabeth has been actively involved with the development of the *Feldenkrais Method* into a respected profession, founding and editing for eighteen years the first *Feldenkrais Journal*, developing educational programs and materials, working with the Practitioner organization, the *Feldenkrais* GUILD, in numerous capacities, and co-founding Feldenkrais Resources with David Zemach-Bersin. Currently she is involved in the training of new Practitioners and recently graduated training groups in Milano, Italy; Biel, Switzerland; and San Diego, California. Elizabeth has maintained an ongoing and varied private practice working with a diverse population including those with severe movement limitations, children, seniors, musicians, and those in chronic pain. She has also worked extensively with athletes, martial artists, and dancers and is known for her ability to apply the Method in dynamic situations. Elizabeth has practiced the martial art of aikido since 1977 and currently holds the rank of sixth degree black belt. (Aikido is a nonviolent martial art centered around neutralizing aggression by redirecting an opponent's force.) Her practice of the *Feldenkrais Method* has been informed and shaped by her experiences in aikido. Elizabeth lives in San Diego, California, with her husband, Rafael Núñez, a professor of cognitive science at the University of California–San Diego, and their daughter.

About David Zemach-Bersin

David Zemach-Bersin is one of Dr. Moshe Feldenkrais's original American students. He studied closely with Dr. Feldenkrais from 1973 to 1984 in the United States, in England, and at the Feldenkrais Institute in Tel Aviv, Israel. He is the co-founder of Feldenkrais Resources and The Feldenkrais Institute of New York. David is the Director of the New York City and the Washington/Baltimore *Feldenkrais Method* Training Programs, and teaches courses for physical and occupational therapists. He is a graduate of UC Berkeley, with extensive post-graduate work in physiological psychology, and is the co-author of *Relaxercise* (HarperCollins), a popular introduction to the *Feldenkrais Method,* as well as the author of many Feldenkrais audio programs. David is the co-founder of the Feldenkrais Research Foundation, a not-for-profit, dedicated to research on Dr. Feldenkrais's ideas. He maintains a private practice in New York and Pennsylvania, working with a diverse population including those with severe movement limitations, chronic pain, and neurological problems, and with world-class musicians and performing artists. David lives with his wife Kaethe, a children's book author and illustrator, in Bucks County, Pennsylvania.

Resources

To find a *Feldenkrais* practitioner in a particular area, or for general information about the *Feldenkrais* Method, contact The *Feldenkrais* Guild, 5436 N. Albina Avenue, Portland, Oregon 97217.

(800) 775-2118 or (503) 221-6612
Website: www.feldenkrais.com

For information regarding *Feldenkrais Method* educational materials that can be used at home, including books, CDs, DVDs, and audio downloads, contact *Feldenkrais* Resources. Walk-in store at 3680 Sixth Avenue, San Diego, California 92103.

(800) 765-1907 or (619) 220-8776
Website: www.feldenkraisresources.com

For information about *Feldenkrais Method* classes, workshops, or the *Feldenkrais* store in Northern California, contact *Feldenkrais* Resources Training Institute, 830 Bancroft Way, Berkeley, California 94710.

(510) 540-7600
Website: www.frtiberkeley.com

For information about *Feldenkrais Method* courses, trainings, and materials on the East Coast, contact The *Feldenkrais* Institute of New York, The Chelsea Arts Building, Second Floor, 134 West 26th Street, New York, New York 10001.

(212) 727-1014
Website: www.feldenkraisinstitute.com

For information on practitioner organizations worldwide, contact the International Feldenkrais Federation.

Website: www.feldenkrais-method.org.

About North Atlantic Books

North Atlantic Books (NAB) is a 501(c)(3) nonprofit publisher committed to a bold exploration of the relationships between mind, body, spirit, culture, and nature. Founded in 1974, NAB aims to nurture a holistic view of the arts, sciences, humanities, and healing. To make a donation or to learn more about our books, authors, events, and newsletter, please visit www.northatlanticbooks.com.